GROW YOUR BABY, NOT YOUR WEIGHT

Durga Shakti Nagpal is a celebrated IAS officer belonging to the Uttar Pradesh cadre. She is known for spearheading the largest crackdown against the notorious sand mafia of the Noida region, an industry worth ₹22,000 crore yearly. Her relentless midnight raids, conducted over a span of several days, are unparalleled in the country's history and were well-lauded. When she was threatened, physically attacked, and hastily removed from her post, there was a national upsurge in her support, and the entire country prayed for her safety. She was on the cover page of national newspapers such as the Times of India and Hindustan Times for several days. The number of times her name was searched on google in a week beat the record held by Sachin Tendulkar at the time. The country wide movement in support of her was seen as a major victory against corruption and the criminalisation of politics. She is also the youngest person to be awarded the Woman of The Year award by the Economic Times.

Durga Shakti is also credited with overhauling the government health and education systems. She has a unique approach to sensitizing and motivating doctors and teachers in government hospitals and schools, which resulted in levels of efficiency that were unheard of in government set-ups.

Her contribution to the environment is exceptional. She undertook a massive plantation drive of 25 lakh plants in a record 7 days, during her tenure in Mathura as Chief Development Officer. What sets her initiative apart is that she accorded highest priority to after-care of the young saplings, through proper and professional watering and manuring.

She has also served as Officer on Special Duty to the Union Agriculture and Farmers Welfare Minister and as Dy CEO of India Brand Equity Foundation, where she propounded Mission Brand India.

Durga Shakti is a motivational speaker, frequently invited to speak by the TED portal and other student communities. Apart from her professional career as an IAS officer, she engages in philanthropic activities regularly, and is a lover of literature, poetry, and fitness. Her motto in life is: Born to Serve.

Her social media handles are @DurgaShaktiIAS on twitter and Durga Shakti Nagpal on LinkedIn. She can also be reached on nagpaldurga@gmail.com

Praise for the book

'If you've been told that motherhood is the end of your career and your youth, you are not alone. Indian women have had to choose between their individuality and having children for too long. Durga Shakti Nagpal's book changes the narrative entirely. A celebrated bureaucrat and a mother of two, Durga shows you how to have it all.'

—Shashi Tharoor
politician, author and former international diplomat

'A power-packed read with enough motivation to fuel you through your pregnancy. The motherhood lodestar we all need.'
—Dr Naresh Trehan
cardiovascular and cardiothoracic surgeon

'A myth-debunking Bible for expecting moms. A two-time mother, Durga sure knows the ropes of a stress-free pregnancy.'
—Hema Malini
actress, dancer and politician

'A must-read for young Indian mothers-to-be, this book by Durga Shakti Nagpal offers the most valuable pregnancy advice.'
—Nitin Gadkari
politician and social entrepreneur

'From a brilliant civil servant and a mother of two, a refreshingly honest take on how to balance work and pregnancy, and the best ways to deal with its unique challenges.'
—Shekhar Gupta
journalist, author and columnist

GROW YOUR BABY, NOT YOUR WEIGHT

An Extraordinary Memoir of Pregnancy, Birthing and Everything Between

DURGA SHAKTI NAGPAL

Published by
Rupa Publications India Pvt. Ltd 2022
7/16, Ansari Road, Daryaganj
New Delhi 110002

Sales Centres:
Allahabad Bengaluru Chennai
Hyderabad Jaipur Kathmandu
Kolkata Mumbai

Copyright © Durga Shakti Nagpal 2022

The views and opinions expressed in this book are the author's own and the facts are as reported by her which have been verified to the extent possible, and the publishers are not in any way liable for the same.

All rights reserved.
No part of this publication may be reproduced, transmitted, or stored in a retrieval system, in any form or by any means, electronic, mechanical, photocopying, recording or otherwise, without the prior permission of the publisher.

ISBN: 978-93-5520-277-2

First impression 2022

10 9 8 7 6 5 4 3 2 1

The moral right of the author has been asserted.

Printed at Gopsons Papers Limited, Noida

This book is sold subject to the condition that it shall not, by way of trade or otherwise, be lent, resold, hired out, or otherwise circulated, without the publisher's prior consent, in any form of binding or cover other than that in which it is published.

*I dedicate my first book to my grandmother,
Mrs Jeewan Bala Mittal, who is a fathomless source of patience,
peace, and perpetual support. She is special as she heads a tribe
of four generations of female members living under one roof!
My pranaam Nani.*

CONTENTS

Foreword by Shilpa Shetty   ix
Acknowledgements   xi
Introduction   xvii

1. Jubilation, Fatigue, Nausea: The Journey Begins   1
2. Enjoying Every Morsel: A Wholesome and Healthy Diet   13
3. Averting the Evidence: Keeping Stretch Marks at Bay   28
4. Sparkle from Within: Glowing Skin   42
5. Weight in Check: Yoga and Walking   51
6. Keep that Spine Straight: Back and Bulge   68
7. Skyrocket Your Energy Level: Second Trimester   80
8. Rediscover Yourself: Final Trimester   90
9. Journey's Finale: Giving Birth   102
10. Same Destination: Different Journeys   113
11. Pregnancy and Child Rearing: It's a Family Affair   125
12. Having it All: A Career and Motherhood Go Hand in Hand   136

FOREWORD

My introduction to the dynamic IAS officer Durga Shakti Nagpal was probably how you may have come to know of her as well: by reading of her exploits in the newspaper. She has had quite an inspiring journey so far. Her achievements amaze me! Knowing her personally feels like I've known her for a long time. She juggles her work and personal life admirably. So, when I learnt that she was penning her pregnancy memoirs, I knew right away that something unique and intriguing was in the works.

Of all the extraordinary experiences from one's life that Durga could have shared with her readers, her chosen subject stood out for me. There are many books about pregnancy experiences, but this was the first one that celebrated the journey itself, without simply focusing on the prize at the end. Durga's is a story of what she saw as the perfect pregnancy experience—not a recovery from pregnancy woes. What is even more special is that Durga's book celebrates a lifelong practice of healthy living, far beyond the pregnancy months alone.

The more I read this book, the more I found myself nodding my head in agreement with what Durga had to say about health and fitness. As a staunch believer of clean eating and healthy living, I have experienced the transformational powers of a good diet and exercise regimen myself. Like me, Durga swears by a lot of traditional remedies and quick fixes, which she fondly calls her *Ma ke Nuskhe*. Science trumps superstition at every point, though, as she takes every trick with a grain of salt and addresses uncomfortable realities of pregnancy and childbirth. She does not pretend that the journey is going to be all milk and honey; in fact, she prepares you for quite the opposite. She acknowledges that there will be pain and distress, and maybe some health scares as well. But she remains adventurous through it all.

'I will never advise anybody to do anything I have not done several times over myself,' she once laughingly told me. It reminds me of the fact that the strength of a woman is her greatest asset.

This book will be one of your most trusted companions throughout the nine months of your pregnancy and even beyond. When you look back on this special time in your life, you will be glad that you chose to pick this up as your pregnancy read.

Shilpa Shetty
actor, entrepreneur and wellness influencer

ACKNOWLEDGEMENTS

Ideas are strange in terms of the routes they take... they spring up out of nowhere and take over your silent meditative minutes, unconsciously distracting you. They are mobile, jumping around the way my 6-year-old daughter Dania does, while you are caught up in an engaging conversation. The idea to write a book sprouted in a similarly confused manner. On a winter's morning, during my early pregnancy (which I call the pinky pregnancy phase), my mother, Mrs. Vinita Nagpal (a devoted homemaker and a treasure trove of hidden charms), was unrelenting in her chatter while we were on a walk. Some stray thought found conception and blossomed into this book. So, my appreciation first goes to my revered mother. Readers will discover that she deserves much more credit than merely seeding this idea. My mother has an almost spiritual ability to conjure up easy recipes at times when my mind is filled with conflicting thoughts!

Joined in coaxing me to write this book was my dear friend, Ravneet Sandhu Guglani, an omni-talented woman with excellent communication skills. She is an entrepreneur and intellectual in her own right. Ravneet was constantly egging me on with her 'misconception' that I am cut out to author bigger treatises. She is thus a clear co-driver for the completion of this book.

This book, which you hold (so lovingly), would not exist but for the willing, encouraging nod that I received from its editorial director, Dibakar Ghosh of Rupa Publications. He gets parallel credit for birthing this project. For much of your reading pleasure, and the clarity and weight of the content, we all owe big thanks to the editing by my dear neighbour, the renowned literary agent Kanishka Gupta, and his associate, the super talented Sunaina Menezes.

I must acknowledge and share two fatherly influences in my life and work. First, my father-in-law, Shri Kripa Shankar Singh, IPS. A 'Karamsheel' in real life, he is a keen observer and thorough disciplinarian. Readers will discern his influence on my daily routine. My own father, Shri Subhash Nagpal, has been the creative inspiration for this work. My earliest memories are that of him scribbling notes for his creative pursuits, notwithstanding his multiple preoccupations. He has taught me to live life to the fullest, instilling and literally injecting in me numerous extracurricular interests. My humour and love for writing thus come easy to me... through inheritance!

My mother-in-law Dr Pramila Singh's constant support

ACKNOWLEDGEMENTS

has been invaluable in my efforts to complete this book while pregnant. She is the gentlest person I have ever known, and you will discover this as you read the book. My gratitude to her for everything is immeasurable. My sister-in-law, Dr Archana Singh, has been my constant source of encouragement in this endeavour. All Dania's fashion goals, and perhaps the ones yet to surface in Digara (our 3-month-old), are inspired by her.

I share my thanks and deep regards to Dr Seema Jain, Max Hospital, for bestowing on me the privilege of being my personal gynaecologist, and a constant companion during my pregnancy, up until the super smooth delivery hour. Dr P.N.V.R. Chengali Rekha, senior gynaecologist at Delhi Cantonment General Hospital, very kindly provided this book with her seasoned medical inputs for the larger benefit of readers. I place Abhishek Singh, my dear husband, in the same category as the doctors, because he is so un-medical in his approach to important health issues, including my pregnancy. His approach—to rely on the inherent intelligence of body and soul for most health irritants—is not only a matter of faith but involves a thorough science of self-healing. Much of my undertakings of growing the child in my womb were guided by his prescriptions, and I have shared this practiced wisdom with my readers as well.

I write about miscellaneous current issues, off and on. Some of you may have come across my write-ups in

English dailies and magazines. Writing a book, however, is a different ballgame altogether. I often say that journeying through pregnancy is a collective affair, and so is creative writing. One owes so much to so many, who brought to the table their varied strengths, from manual support to inventive inputs. First in this series is Urbi Chatterjee, who, through her ready availability for frequent chats, ever-evolving vocabulary, and ingenious prose, provided hearty support in this venture. I cherish this association and wish her success in her future endeavours. I applaud Prof Ghazala Naaz, a passionate teacher of English language and literature, for sustaining an active interest in women in contemporary literature and history, and for painstakingly going through my manuscript. She pointed out some overlooked flaws, with her eagle eye precision and mastery of English grammar, and offered appropriate and subtle changes.

I owe my personal physical and mental fitness to two main sources. For the right body weight, balance, fighting fitness, and rhythm I owe a great deal to my fitness trainer Jugal Kishore. My motto through pregnancy, particularly my second pregnancy, was to achieve and sustain the state of what I call 'Pregnant Fit'. For ensuring success in this mission, I also raise a herbal and yogic toast to Mrs. Sushila Biswas, a mother of two and a most capable and disciplined yoga instructor. She insists that I have 'worked very hard

ACKNOWLEDGEMENTS

to get lucky'. Images of the Yogic postures that you see in the book are professionally captured by Sumit Sahni in a very clear and comprehensive manner. His pictures bring authenticity to my training sessions, and I am sure they will inspire lots of moms-to-be in their blissful journey through pregnancy.

Rajan Prajapati has been my Man Friday, my right-hand man since I met him in 2015. This book landed in his lap, repeatedly, for various solutions. His Midas touch produced pure gold (as far as I know). Mozzam Ali Khan Afridi who takes care of my office is our one-man army. He single-handedly solves all problems under the sun! With him around, I could focus all my energies on writing this book. My mobility to and from my government office, my pursuit of extracurricular interests during my advancing pregnancy, and the rigmarole of writing, fitness sessions, and, of course, visits to the hospital, were made smooth thanks to my chauffeur, Ajay Kumar Tripathi. Thank you, my man. I wish you good health and familial happiness.

I thank my dear readers for choosing to pick up this book, with faith in its utility and reading satisfaction. I invite you to offer your feedback, as well as suggestions for the benefit of future moms, whereby they can enrich and enjoy their pregnancy voyage. I also invite those of you who wish to translate this work into other languages, should you find it useful. At the same time, I request you to please spread the word and the positive message of the book amongst your real and virtual fraternity.

In concluding this rather long note of acknowledgement, I sincerely and wholeheartedly convey my gratitude to all the famous celebrities who put their stamp of approval on this work. Their individual stature of being great achievers, performers, and giant intellectuals cast an aura of sunshine upon this work.

I am tempted to end with the quote 'Happiness is... carrying a whole world inside you'. Acknowledging this message's energizing appeal, I urge all future moms to practice such affirmation in their nine-month sojourn full of happiness-agony-euphoria. May you sparkle from within! Bon voyage...

INTRODUCTION

When we are born into this world, we bring with us an intuitive sense of wonder. Babies and toddlers explore the world with great gusto. For them, every discovery holds a wonderful fascination be it mummy's face, a spoon, or even an unusually shaped piece of rock. They have a deep connection to the magic that is intrinsic to this planet and its occupants. As we grow older, we begin to lose this tenuous thread. With age, life makes us a bit jaded at times, and our innate sense of wonder can get buried underneath the everyday mundanity of survival.

There comes a time in one's life when one begins a unique journey of creation, the creation of a new human life. This is our chance to reconnect with that old sense of awe, a reawakening of the magic of our life. Childbirth is the closest that one can come to touching perfection. It is the fruition of a miraculous coming together of body and soul. Having had the incredible fortune of experiencing the joy of motherhood, not once but twice, I have come to

Grow Your Baby, Not Your Weight

recognise pregnancy for what it truly is—God's greatest gift to humankind. I have tried to tread this path with dignity and grace, drinking in every moment of joy and toil, and I have learnt a thing or two in the process. I hope, my dear reader, to serve as your friend and companion through this book, on this miraculous road to motherhood, and to provide the support that every mother-to-be so desperately needs from a fellow sister.

Advanced medicine and scientific progress have made many areas of life—traditionally fraught with danger—easy and routine. But in some cases, this has had a detrimental impact as well, making natural processes appear much more complex than they really are. Pregnancy and childbirth are prime examples. While modern medical knowledge has greatly reduced the dangers to mother and child, heightened medical scrutiny has made the journey to childbirth far too technical, pushing a perfectly natural phenomenon into the zone of a medical condition! Mothers-to-be today are inundated with advice, suggestions, and cautionary tales about the many restrictions they now have to incorporate into their own lives. Let me tell you right away, you are not in a state of critical medical emergency! You will have a baby. Congratulations, and welcome to the most rewarding journey of your life. Now get up and get going. Live your life the way you always have—if anything, work on discovering the improved version of yourself. We mothers-to-be have

Introduction

to guard against letting the world bring us down. Take it from me, you are not indisposed. Respect your doctor's directions, especially in case of a complex pregnancy. But for the rest of it, don't let any kind of fears get to you.

More often than not, we fail to acknowledge the enormous role that our minds play in guiding our lives. A big part of the human experience takes place inside the mind, so it is vital to hone the mind in a manner that serves you best. I strongly believe that the key to this is focus and discipline. Your mind should be your greatest ally in life, and not a deterrent to your goals. Focus and discipline are muscles that need to be strengthened, and these go a long way in determining your experience during pregnancy. Grit and resilience will be your best friends, as will an unwavering focus on your ultimate goal—the arrival of your child. The path will not always be quite as easy as you would like, and this is when your mental muscles will come to your aid.

My own course in life led me to build my focus and bolster my discipline from an early age. Being from a family of bureaucrats, I knew from a young age that that was the life I wanted for myself. I aspired for the upper echelons of government service. I never harboured illusions about the effort that I needed to put in to make my dream a reality. I started casually perusing study materials for the Civil Services examinations from the time I was in high school. By the time college commenced, I had already gained an initiation into the gruelling process of preparation. I studied Engineering in Delhi while staying in a hostel, as my father was posted in Lucknow at the time. Anyone who has stayed in a hostel knows that time and energy come at a premium there. One has to look after all sorts of household chores—cleaning, washing, and basic housekeeping—while also attending classes, maintaining good grades, and enjoying life as a young person. I was determined not to miss out on the opportunities that college life had to offer, but at the same time, my mind was fixed on a singular goal—the train to Mussoorie, where all new IAS (Indian Administrative Service) recruits started their careers at the Lal Bahadur Shastri National Academy of Administration (LBSNAA). I made it a point to put aside a few hours of study time every single day for the preparation of the civil service examination, even as I juggled the quintessential college life.

After four fruitful years, I graduated as a Computer Science engineer with good grades and two cushy job offers from prestigious companies in hand. As a twenty-one-year-old, fresh off the boat, straining for financial independence and the opportunity to forge my way ahead in life, I found myself in the midst of a major dilemma. I did not want to give up the opportunity to work and earn, but I had still not lost sight of my ultimate goal of joining the Services. I turned to my father for advice, and as always, his reassuring

Introduction

words aided me in my decision. My father reminded me of a fundamental rule to achieve anything significant in life. He told me that I could not afford to have a Plan B. 'You will get jobs again, if you need them. Right now, though, it is time for you to take the plunge and prepare for the examination. Give yourself a year; no more, and no less. And tell yourself that at the end of it, you should have an offer from UPSC in hand. Make a decision, and see it through, no matter what.'

Indeed, I saw it through. I dedicated eighteen hours daily to my studies, allocating the remaining time for basic needs of existence. I brought two sets of pyjamas with me that I could alternate between, having sworn not to buy myself a new set until I received my offer letter! Towards the end of the year, these pyjama sets started resembling rags, pale and torn as they were. There came a point when my mother refused to repair these any longer—the eighth time, according to her, was just about enough. But I stuck to my guns—no new clothes for me before I reached my goal. I had made a commitment to myself, and I was going to honour it, come what may. So, there I was, armed with discipline, focus, and a couple of shoddy pyjamas, determined to win. I was not disappointed—an All India Rank of 20 made the punishing regime worth every minute of it. My father, having learnt the news of the results from a friend while at a game of golf, shed a few tears of pride. His daughter had achieved what she had set her mind to, and he was proud.

Courage and determination have also been my loyal companions in life. They have helped me achieve new heights, both professionally and personally. As a young officer at her first deputation as an SDM, I came up against the deadly sand mafia network of Noida. These organised criminals were involved in illegal sand mining, an operation that had a far-reaching impact on the lives of the local villagers as well as the environment and the government treasury. After being approached by the helpless farmers suffering as a result of flooding of embankments and a subsequent loss of home and livelihood, I decided to take this devilish enterprise by the horns. I organised midnight raids, maintaining absolute secrecy, and started making dents in their illegal empire. The sand mafia had resources, and traveled in cavalcades of SUVs, while we had to function with restricted manpower and decrepit vehicles. After a few weeks of continued raiding, threats were issued against us. By this time, though, we had shaken up the foundations of a hitherto untouched empire, and slowly but surely, the walls began to crumble. A few weeks into the project, we succeeded in arresting over a hundred people and gathering royalty worth several crore rupees for the government treasury. We brought the fearsome mining empire to its knees, an unprecedented achievement. The gratitude the

Introduction

villagers expressed by the end of it made all the risks and the threats to life and safety worth it. Courage had seen my team and me through, and we had emerged victorious.

But what do any of these have to do with pregnancy and motherhood, you ask? Well, life teaches you how to deal with every situation flung at you—you just have to recognise lessons for what they are. My professional preparation and achievements taught me the life skills necessary to tackle the journey that is being a parent. They trained my mind and prepared it for endurance and dogged perseverance, and the ability to conquer fear—qualities that one needs every step of the way in the pregnancy journey. My life taught me to take on pregnancy as I would any other crucial project, and to employ the same strategies of planning and preparation to deal with every step of the journey.

I have aimed for perfection in every area of my life—I always feel that anything worth doing is worth doing well. The first time I was expecting a child, I was able to treat my life as a laboratory for best practices. The second time, my ideas were proved beyond doubt. There were little tweaks in my approach for my second pregnancy—particularly in terms of my mental and emotional health, which I had not been entirely conscious of the first time around. This taught me the importance of forgiving oneself for one's lapses and getting up to give it another go. And it strengthened my confidence in my tribe. There is nothing that a woman cannot achieve if she puts her heart and soul to it.

Every step of my journey would have been incomplete without the untiring support of my husband Abhishek Singh, my companion, my special person. He is an IAS officer and an actor, and it is his bottomless wellspring of enthusiasm in life, his energy, and his willingness to take the plunge that keeps me going. Abhishek is my inspiration in how he makes the most of every minute of his life, participating in all his passions—from bureaucracy to fashion, from acting to social work, and of course, parenting—with an ever-increasing enthusiasm.

This is my story of living a happy pregnancy. I am breastfeeding my baby now, and I rarely get more than two hours of sleep at a time. But hey, it could have been even less! Sleep deprived, overextended, and exhausted as I am, I have never been happier or more fulfilled in my life. And I wish nothing less for you. This is my way of nudging you along on that journey.

In this book, I will walk you through the journey of pregnancy in intimate detail. You will get to experience pregnancy as I did, with the advantage of wisdom in hindsight. Spread over twelve chapters, we will delve into every minute aspect of life during those nine months, and the months beyond. We will start where it all begins: the breaking of the 'good news', the astonishment and anticipation, followed, far too quickly, by the dreaded nausea

Introduction

of early pregnancy. But there are ways to beat this ugly monster at its own game—and I shall show you exactly how I did it.

In the next four chapters, we will explore the crucial facets of pregnant life: diet and exercise, skin and stretch marks, weight gain and spinal pressure. There is much to be said when it comes to these arenas, but not everything one hears is worth practicing. I will give you an insight into the habits, the routines, and the hacks that allowed me to stay fighting fit throughout the trimesters. Age-old advice must be remodelled to suit the needs of the modern woman with a hectic life—as I did. You get a glimpse into my pregnancy rituals, some of my favourite recipes, and tricks that I swear by.

When it comes to diets, our focus will remain on maintaining balance and not falling for fads. It is important to put thought and care into the meals we consume, as much as it is recommended that we find joy in eating. The act of eating can become meditative, spiritual even, if done with the right mindset: this is what we shall strive to cultivate during pregnancy.

Our skin, the largest organ of our bodies, faces much discomfort at this stage. And yet our skin does a lot of the talking in public, impacting our standing in society, whether we like it or not. And so, we will give it the attention that is its due in our journey. From tracking stretch marks to eating skin-friendly food, I will share it all.

The importance of a consistent, well-regulated workout routine cannot be overstated in the context of pregnancy—but also in life as a whole. There are many misconceptions and myths surrounding the safety of physical exertion for an expecting mother. As a habitual workout fanatic, I shall share my experience of the positive impact that sweat and movement have had on me. Be it in maintaining the ideal weight during pregnancy, preventing avoidable aches and pains, or even ensuring quality of skin—far too much is linked to the issue of weight and exercise. And so, I have gone into painstaking detail about the overwhelming influence that exercising wields in this phase of life.

The experiences of an expecting mother change with each trimester, and I have tried to capture my own journey through these phases. We will explore the blessing that is trimester two and look at ways that our energies can be harnessed to work at their peak during this time. We will move on to the final trimester and all the anticipation, tinged with apprehension, it inevitably brings. And so, we shall reach the final leg, all the way to the day of reckoning, when a battle of will against body finally brings the baby into our arms.

There are other equally significant aspects of pregnancy that sometimes get overlooked because they happen to be less physiological and more psychological. I will talk about the

Introduction

important relationships in my life, and the people without whose consistent support my journey would have been far more strenuous. It is an important reminder that childbirth and motherhood are not accomplished in isolation and are in fact joint ventures for the community. I shall explore the importance of maintaining one's own life and identity as a mother, and how I was able to achieve a balance between parenting and career obligations. And finally, I shall reflect upon my two experiences of pregnancy, and the commonalities and variations I faced on these occasions.

While a big part of this book revolves around my personal experiences, philosophies, and outlook on life, I strongly affirm the universality of much of this journey. Being a mother twice over has made my life complete in a sense that I had not been aware was possible. I wish the same joy and fulfillment for you, dear reader. It is my honour to take this journey with you. Happy birthing!

1

JUBILATION, FATIGUE, NAUSEA: THE JOURNEY BEGINS

Fairy tales typically open with princesses and enchanted forests, talking animals and ancient curses. Mine began with a feeling of uneasiness, followed by an early morning visit to the loo and two little pink lines on a pregnancy test stick! Two little lines that I had been eagerly awaiting, but I still felt overwhelmed when they did appear.

Let me tell you a little secret about pregnancy: it's surreal!

The sense of immense exhilaration that washes over you is difficult to adequately describe in words. Pregnancy is perhaps the closest that human beings can get to the power of creation. And only the female of the species has this ability. Take a moment to let that sink in. A pregnant woman is often said to be in a 'delicate' condition. Delicate? I felt ready to take on the world without a single hair on my head out of place. I had never felt so much in control of my body. A pregnant woman is a true force of nature, so be careful not to tick her off!

Finding out that you are pregnant is a study in the complexity of the human mind. Even as I basked in my new-found sense of power, my brain went into overdrive. A new member of the family was on its way. Suddenly, all I could see in the room around me was clutter. We needed to make space. My new identity would be Durga Shakti, Master Space Creator. My body was well ahead of me, busily creating a comfortable and nourishing first home for this new little guest for nine months. I needed to make sure that it had all the space required later as well, when the baby was out in the world. A cleaning spree was evidently in order.

> **Dr Rekha on routine tests and screenings:** In cases where a woman approaches a doctor prior to conception, screening for certain underlying conditions are advised such as epilepsy, anaemia, heart diseases, etc. which are a cause for concern in terms of the mother or baby's health. These conditions are then treated or controlled before planning a pregnancy. When the woman has already conceived, certain routine tests are conducted, such as a complete

Jubilation, Fatigue, Nausea: The Journey Begins

> blood profile, random blood sugar and viral markers, blood grouping and typing, etc. as broad screening for infections and diseases. Periodic ultrasounds are also conducted at specific intervals throughout the pregnancy to monitor the health and development of the baby.

The first obvious step was to inform my husband, Abhishek. I knew that this was going to be a highly interesting experience. I could hardly wait to see his reaction.

Abhishek and I had had 'the talk' just a month before this. We had both agreed that Dania, our 5-year-old daughter, needed a sibling. It was the ideal time for us to try for another baby. And less than a month later, here I was, waving the stick of joy in his face.

'Are you *absolutely* sure?' he asked me for the third time, pacing about the room excitedly.

There was a look of wonder on his face. 'Uh, two pink lines... that means positive, right?' He continued to be amazed at how this had happened so soon after we decided on having our second child.

'You know *na*, that home kits are not a hundred percent foolproof? You should visit the doctor so we can confirm this.' (I took his advice, but the doctor also asked me to come back after three weeks with the first ultrasound.)

This sense of joy and disbelief was going to last for a while—for two entire months, as it turned out! Though I had already given birth once before, the sense of wonder struck me all over again. What was this miracle of life, in which a speck inside my body was going to transform into a strapping human, maybe several feet tall, one day? Abhishek and I were thrilled.

But there would be plenty of time to philosophise later. Now, on to action.

The news was yet to be delivered (pardon the pun) to the most important person.

I found Her Highness in the garden, playing fetch with the dog. 'Dania, come here. I want to tell you a secret.'

She came running at once, always eager to 'share the tea'. I knelt down to whisper conspiratorially into her ear, 'Do you know, you are about to be a big sister. Mumma Papa are getting a little sibling for you.'

Dania listened with an excited face. Then she looked me in the eye and said, 'Please get me a sister. I don't think I want a little boy.'

I laughed and told her that I would keep her request in mind, and she nodded contentedly before returning to her games. And for a moment, I thought that was that. But if you have ever met a precocious five-year old, you would know that they have an unlimited ability to take you by surprise.

I had just sat down to begin the day's work when Dania came running into the room. 'Mumma, I told chotu bhaiya

Jubilation, Fatigue, Nausea: The Journey Begins

that you are getting me a little sister.'

I did a double take. 'You told him *what?*'

'Please don't be angry, I know you said that this was a secret. But chotu bhaiya will not tell anyone else, I promise!'

I soon found out that my five-year-old had in fact taken up the responsibility of being my media handler, announcing the news of my pregnancy more efficiently than a press release to the national dailies! She had told her grandparents as well as other family members, telling them that this was a big secret and asking them to promise that they would not tell mumma about it. My in-laws looked at me askance, unsure about whether to take this announcement seriously, seeing that it had come from a child.

For a while, things continued to be quite awkward for Abhishek and me. In Indian households, traditionally, the news that a woman is expecting is shared with the family only after three months. But when you have a trailblazing daughter, it can be difficult to maintain such norms. Eventually, we agreed to include the entire family in our secret, just so we could start looking each other in the eye again!

Pregnancy is all fun and games until the fatigue sets in. One day, you wake up with your body feeling unbelievably heavy. It is as if an invisible boulder has been attached to you, and you have to drag its weight with you everywhere you go. This is a very strange feeling, and most recurrent in the first trimester of the pregnancy. The body has an entirely new and incredibly important role to play—it is getting ready to create a new human being. Suddenly, all systems in your body automatically start working overtime. The heart pumps your blood at a rate heightened by almost twenty percent, sending it in streams to make your womb safe and comfortable for your baby. So, while the tiredness can be bothersome, it is in fact an indication of the many rapid, crucial changes that are taking place inside your body.

I spent these days with a permanent feeling of drowsiness. Sometimes, I would feel my eyes drooping in the middle of the workday. A sense of constant exhaustion accompanied me round the clock. Although I was sleeping longer than usual, I would wake up feeling tired. This was a strange time for me. One expects pregnancy to follow a linear curve, with each month being progressively more difficult than the previous ones, and with the first trimester being an easy trial period. But this misconception was quickly dispelled. This was going to be a bumpy ride, in more ways than one!

This was a time that I spent marveling at the power and adaptability of my own body. Truly, the female body is a miracle. It is like a highly complex computer with intricate functions, but unlike the machines built by human science, the body draws its power from a much older, more primal source: Nature itself. Its power to learn from cues and to adapt accordingly are unparalleled.

Jubilation, Fatigue, Nausea: The Journey Begins

With each passing day, I could feel my body moulding itself to fit the changing circumstances, making itself more and more equipped to deal with my current needs. Soon, it seemed that my body was reading my mind, and adjusting its state in order to help me defeat the lethargy and imminent drowsiness, and spring back into action instead.

The first real test of pregnancy sets in at about the end of the first month. Yes, you guessed it right, this is the proverbial 'morning sickness', Bollywood's favourite indicator of a potentially dubious state of motherhood for the heroine. But unlike in the movies, it does not do you the courtesy of limiting itself to one session in the morning. No ma'am, you had better get used to a new state of being, with your day revolving around your nauseous or dizzy spells.

For the blissfully uninitiated, let me try to fill you in on this special part of the child-bearing journey. Think of how it feels when you have a stomach bug—there is a churning sensation in your stomach, your head spins, and the world seems unsteady. Suddenly, you seem to be made of some turbulent, jelly-like material, and all you want to do is stick your head over the chamber pot and throw your guts up. You hope that this will ease the sensation—and sometimes it does. But other times, the dizziness continues even though you can feel that your insides have emptied out. For the next few months, until the fourth or perhaps the fifth month, this is going to be your frequent daily routine. Bizarre, is it not?

The term morning sickness is slightly misleading. The fact is, nausea and dizziness may continue intermittently throughout the day. It could even be triggered by certain smells, including the aroma of food that once used to be your favourite.

> **Dr Rekha on nausea:** The most common problem that almost all women face during pregnancy is nausea and vomiting (morning sickness). The cause of nausea is the increased levels of a hormone in the body called human chorionic gonadotropin (HCG) or the pregnancy hormone. However, nausea can be managed by taking small, frequent meals instead of three meals in a day. One can also have dry toast in the morning soon after waking up. Those who experience excessive nausea can take the support of medication to control it.

This is when you start exerting your full mental prowess. Pregnancy, as with so many of life's challenges, is won or lost by the power of the mind. When you are in firm control of your thoughts and emotions, you can wield your mind in order to overcome most difficulties. During this period, I concentrated all my energy into harnessing my willpower and my patience. I knew that I would not

Jubilation, Fatigue, Nausea: The Journey Begins

let this inconvenience throw my days into disarray. It was time to put into practice all my years of self-management and mindset training. I was confident that the 'labour' and perseverance I had practiced, first, in preparation for the civil services, and then, my victory over the trials and tribulations I faced as an IAS officer, would surely pave the way for a smooth labour, yet again.

I sailed through this phase of my pregnancy. I was incredibly lucky, but it was not passive luck that propped me up. It was luck manifested through mental control. I chose not to give in to the temporary physical duress, focusing instead on my experience as a whole.

There was a golden rule that I abided by at every turn—nobody knows my body as intimately as I do, and so, I am best placed to make the most appropriate decisions for it. Of course, this is not to say that you should go against your doctor's express instructions. But as all mothers-to-be know only too well, this is a time when everyone around has suggestions and advice about how best to conduct yourself. I lent a polite ear to everyone but stuck to my own instincts and self-knowledge while making decisions about what worked best for me.

The most sustainable way in which you can devise a plan of action for yourself is through rigorous trial and error. What a certain person finds soothing might heighten somebody else's nausea.

Grow Your Baby, Not Your Weight

Eventually, though, I was able to narrow down a few things that worked like magic. The age-old lemon and honey in warm water, first thing in the morning, did wonders to soothe my nausea. The smell of lemon was an added benefit—the citrusy scent helped with the overall queasiness in my oestrogen-fueled body.

Another fun trick that helped me during this time was tracking my nausea clock. For most pregnant women, there are certain times of the day, or even during the morning, when nausea hits with full force. But it can help to beat morning sickness at its own game. I quickly noticed that I tended to feel the worst when I woke up, at around 6 am. I had to rush to the bathroom immediately and began my days with a rancid taste in my mouth. I resolved to try waking up a little earlier the next day. Immediately after leaving the bed, I got myself out of the house for a quick stroll. The cool morning breeze felt heavenly on my face. The fresh air made me feel energized and ready to tackle the day ahead. I came back home after a leisurely walk of thirty minutes, and just as I had expected, I did not feel at all nauseous. The train of morning sickness had missed its station and decided to leave me behind that day.

Walking also solved the problem of working out. During the first trimester of pregnancy, doctors advise against all forms of exercise, even mild ones like yoga. But walking is a good alternative that remains a safe option throughout pregnancy.

Jubilation, Fatigue, Nausea: The Journey Begins

I enjoyed my morning walk immensely, and it took me no time at all to make this a daily habit, one that I have continued long after my pregnancy was over. Looking back, I sometimes wonder whether morning sickness had really been a blessing in disguise, allowing me to incorporate a healthy, lifelong habit. Since my childhood, my father has often quoted a German philosopher who said that 'if you keep walking, everything will be alright.' Meaning that all your problems would be resolved. I had agreed with his philosophical message before, but now I could appreciate its value in literal terms.

I also made it a point to keep drinking water throughout the day. Hydration is vital at any given point of time, but its importance cannot be overstated during pregnancy. Water keeps nausea at bay and helps beat sleepiness and even exhaustion. Just remember, almost two-thirds of your body consists of water, and now that your body is working so much harder to create another human, keeping the water levels replenished is your supreme duty. It is the fuel, together with oxygen and food, which keep you running and your baby growing.

Fruits as snacks help mitigate nausea too. My personal favourite is the banana—rich in potassium, fiber, and antioxidants, it is as tasty as it is nutritious. If you tire of eating fruit by itself, a quick dash of rock salt and a spritz of lemon can transform most humble fruits into a gourmet

Grow Your Baby, Not Your Weight

meal. You want to keep your meals small but frequent. A stomach filled to its brim is not your friend. In fact, I started to eat slightly less than I usually did, just to be on the safe side. Frequent, light meals chewed slowly into its most digestible form help keep your stomach happy. Ensure that the gaps in between meals don't stretch too long, though, otherwise the acids in your stomach will go to work on the lining itself, causing you to make a beeline for the loo.

And finally, don't forget to talk to your mother. I was truly fortunate to have my mother's *Ma ke Nuskhe* while dealing with pregnancy. My mother insisted that I have chaach with chia seeds. I was uncertain about this combination, until a sip left me smacking my lips and then craving more. This light curd and water drink works wonders for cooling the stomach, and the chia seeds provide the much-required fiber to help with digestion, because lest you forget, constipation is another of your lovely companions at this time!

As I adjusted to all the changes happening in my body, and consequently, to my life, I made it a priority to keep a positive outlook. Every time I felt anxiety or doubt creeping up on me, I reminded myself of the primary reason for experiencing everything that I was: I was making a baby, and I would do whatever it took to keep my child healthy and fit.

2

ENJOYING EVERY MORSEL: A WHOLESOME AND HEALTHY DIET

They say that you are what you eat. I have no bones to pick with this advice, but I think this is only a part of the story. You are *what* you eat, but also *when, how,* and *how much*. The anatomy of a good eating habit has at least these many components. And never does this adage become more crucial to your everyday wellbeing than when you are expecting.

As an expecting mother, I felt all sorts of emotions that ultimately made my tummy growl. A routine for eating had to be drawn up, one that would please my tongue, my gut, and my heart simultaneously. I quickly developed a newfound sense of respect for nutritionists. The time and effort that is spent on figuring out the right kind of meal plan is no joking matter.

It is vital that the meals we consume make us happy. Far too often, 'healthy' food turns out to be bland and tasteless. As a pregnant, vegetarian woman, several people suggested that I incorporate boiled dal in my diet as a nutritious snack. Swearing by my trial-and-error rule, I decided to give it a shot. The sight of the boiled dal sitting in a bowl made me sad, but I went ahead and finished the bowl regardless. I'm glad that I did, because it made the decision-making process easy: I was never going to put myself through that ordeal again, even if I were paid to do it. The experiment had been a clear failure.

After the failed experiment, my immediate reaction was wanting to eat shahi paneer for the entirety of the next week. It does not take a doctor to realise that this is a bad idea at any point, but downright dangerous for a pregnant lady. In fact, I probably would not have enjoyed several consequent meals of shahi paneer. By the third meal, I am sure I would have been sick of the very sight of the rich, creamy dish.

The essence of eating well is that it is only effective if we can do it consistently. And this can only be achieved when you plan your meals in such a manner that you look forward to eating each one. Essentially, your meals have to

Enjoying Every Morsel: A Wholesome and Healthy Diet

fall somewhere between the two extremes of bland dal and creamy paneer! Remember: 'nutritious' does not need to be bland. These meals should make you happy; the food should make you want to get out of bed in the morning and look forward to lunchtime. I believe this should be the true meaning of 'comfort food'—food that keeps you thoroughly satisfied and well-nourished.

It was with these guidelines in mind that I set out to create my own menu. I was already having warm water with lemon and honey first thing in the morning, as it helped with my nausea. Now, after doing some research, I decided to add alkaline food to my breakfast. We have all heard of cosmetic material having different pH levels, ranging from acidic to basic (or alkaline).

Our blood, too, has a pH value of its own, slightly over 7, making it a little on the alkaline side. With the pregnancy-induced increase in blood flow, it is useful to adjust our food intake in a manner that bolsters the blood's natural balance.

Uncooked foods—particularly fresh fruits and vegetables—have an alkaline pH value and are a good option to start your day with. In fact, let's face it, it is unlikely that you can overdo your consumption of greens. Think back to your childhood: wasn't your mother constantly asking you to finish your sabzi? I know mine was. As a mother myself, and an expecting one, I made it my duty to ensure that both my babies got adequate vitamins and minerals from leafy veggies and fruits, be that through their own meals or through mine.

Pregnancy takes a toll on the digestive system. Hormonal changes in the body cause the digestive muscles to relax and slow down. Everything becomes more difficult to digest than usual, including your long-time staples. This is something you have to constantly keep in mind while eating. With all the aches, cramps, and nausea you are already feeling, you do not want to add constipation to the mix, if you can help it.

Fresh greens fit in well with my sustainable, happiness-based diet, while also providing roughage and alkali. I decided to experiment as much as I could with salads. The beauty of salads is that you are restricted only by your own imagination. You can toss up a variety of absolutely delicious combinations with staples like cucumber, tomatoes, and carrots. Sprouts add the perfect blend of crunchiness. Simply soak your raw moong dal (green gram lentil) overnight, drain the water the next morning and keep them covered in a sieve until the evening. Voila! You have your own fresh sprouts ready to be eaten. For my sprout salads, I stick to light dressing choices like lemon juice, honey, olive oil, and sprinkled herbs like basil to add a little tang. This is your chance to put your kitchen garden mixes to good use. It is best to steer clear of thick, creamy dressings like

Enjoying Every Morsel: A Wholesome and Healthy Diet

mayonnaise that are unnecessarily heavy on the stomach. Grocery stores offer a wide range of light salad dressings for different occasions, so you never need to run out of new flavours.

The possibilities with fresh vegetables are endless. As Indians, we are blessed to be given the choice of over thirty different cuisines, all of which offer multiple ways to prepare fresh, local vegetables. The emphasis is on the word 'local' here. Over and above burning a hole into your pocket, exotic, frozen celery in the middle of a North Indian summer will have much lower nutritional value compared to the easily available local beans and greens. And, in case you are living away from your native place, this is a great time to try out locally grown ingredients. Let the seasons be your ally in your quest to eat and live healthy.

This is not to say that you cannot experiment with other cuisines. If you are due for a summer birth, green soups and vegetable stews with different seasonings are perfect for your winter pregnancy. Give your mind free reign and experiment with humble staples—that is exactly what I did. I grew up eating (and disliking) daliya. It comes close to the bland, boiled lentils on my list of melancholic foods. But since I already had a lot of vegetables chopped up for all the salads I was making, I decided to try different combinations of veggie daliya. Once I had tasted the result, there was no going back. In fact, I am proud to announce that vegetable daliya with fresh winter veggies like carrots, beans, broccoli, zucchini, and baby corn has now become a favourite evening snack for the entire family.

When it comes to non-vegetarian food, once again, it becomes a matter of moderation. Our most popular meat and fish dishes tend to be rich in oil and spices. Butter chicken and rogan josh, laalmaas and fish kaliya, mutton kosha and biryani—a delight for the tongue but a burden for the tummy. These dishes don't do you any favours during pregnancy, and if one is being truthful, they should be consumed in limited quantities even otherwise. But this does not have to mean turning vegetarian for nine long months. Not at all! There are just as many healthy non-vegetarian dishes as there are vegetarian ones. Grill your fish and chicken, smoke or barbecue your kebabs (no deep frying your shami and galaouti kebabs) and have them with sautéed vegetables. Steam your fish and give East Asian food a run for its money. Try various chicken soup styles. It is actually easier to ensure adequate protein intake during pregnancy as a meat-eater. So, count your blessings and bring out your cookbooks and your inner Masterchef. The rogan josh will weigh you down, but the lightly cooked dishes will keep your 'josh' high throughout the pregnancy.

But just as you are rolling up your sleeves and jumping headlong into your pregnancy-fuelled culinary adventure, it is important to remember one golden rule: pregnancy is

Enjoying Every Morsel: A Wholesome and Healthy Diet

not an excuse to give up on fitness goals. On the contrary, with the right kind of eating and exercise regimen, this can actually become the time when you finally achieve the weight loss (or gain) goals that you have always wished for. It is a myth that pregnancy is a time for weight gain. It should be only 'belly' weight gain, and this is attainable by eating and exercising right.

A very popular common myth about pregnancy is that you have to eat for two people. Please don't believe these stories! Your walnut-sized embryo does *not* need you to eat four slices of pizza and a whole plate of chole bhature. In reality, pregnant women do not require more food than their usual intake, except in the last trimester. The famous Japanese teaching 'hara hachi bun me' says eat until you are 80 percent full for a slim and healthy body. This applies even during pregnancy and therefore it is recommended that you eat slightly less during this time too. Keep your tummy from being overfull. Just as a full bottle of water cannot churn water, so a saturated stomach finds it much tougher to grind your food down.

Sudden pangs of hunger are a common problem during pregnancy. There were times when, in the middle of a work meeting, all I could think about was my packed lunch box back in my office. Such distractions make it difficult to focus on work and lead to unnecessary snacking. It is this sort of snacking that leads to unnecessary weight gain. It is crucial that you train your mind not to give in to these cravings. At the same time, keep having small frequent meals to prevent your stomach from becoming empty. Pregnancy is a time when one is most susceptible to picking up a habit of overeating. If you double the number of rotis you have during a craving-fueled meal, chances are that you will stop being satisfied with your usual number of rotis in the future as well. Eventually, the increased intake will become the norm, and your fitness goals will be much harder to achieve.

Pregnancy is a magical time, and though the nine months can sometimes feel infinitely stretched out, they actually pass you by in the blink of an eye. I reminded myself to constantly savour every moment of my journey, even the more uncomfortable ones. And I carried forward this same attitude of mindfulness when it came to what I ate. I learned to listen to my body and honour its needs. The body has a very efficient alarm clock that informs you about hunger, thirst, and exhaustion. I consciously paid attention to this feeling in my stomach while eating and stopped while there was still some space left in it. It was often annoying and frustrating to have to stop before I felt full, but this temporary irritation was more than adequately compensated for by the feeling of lightness and energy I retained through the rest of the day.

However, even with the best of intentions and the most

Enjoying Every Morsel: A Wholesome and Healthy Diet

efficiently planned systems, we are still human. Despite trying not to, we *will* end up snacking. There will be celebrations and social gatherings, work difficulties and fights with family members. And we *will* turn to food for comfort. So, it is best to account for such inevitabilities and concentrate on snacking right.

As Indians, we are notorious for our love of hot beverages. Be it tea or coffee, it is not unusual for us to have several cups a day. Even though healthier options like green tea and decaffeinated coffee are widely available, we seldom opt for them, sticking to our creamy, milky pleasures instead. Unfortunately, many women have a difficult time digesting milk during pregnancy, and I was no different. My guilty pleasure is masala chai, and in no way was I giving it up for nine long months, health concerns be damned. So, I came up with my own special recipe that didn't disturb my stomach at all and I could continue drinking it throughout my pregnancy. It's so simple to make and has a wonderful taste and aroma.

MAKING YOUR FAVORITE MASALA CHAI AND CHAI MASALA

Ingredients required for approximately 120 g of chai masala powder:
1. Green cardamom – 40 g
2. Black pepper – 50 g
3. Dry ginger – 20 g
4. Cinnamon sticks – 30 g
5. Cloves – 10 g
6. Nutmeg – 2 in nos.
7. Dry tulsi leaves – 6 g/20 leaves (optional)
8. Saffron – 2 g (optional)

Method of preparation:
1. Take a pan and dry roast all the ingredients over a low flame till you start getting an aromatic smell. This will take approximately 3-4 mins.
2. Let this mixture cool till it comes down to room temperature.
3. Grind it coarsely in a blender.
4. Store it in a small airtight container to keep the fragrance intact.

Ingredients for one cup of masala tea:
1. Water – ¾ cup
2. Your homemade chai masala powder – 1 pinch

Enjoying Every Morsel: A Wholesome and Healthy Diet

3. Tea leaves – ¾ teaspoon
4. Milk – ¼ cup
5. Sugar to taste

Method of preparation:

1. Boil the water and add tea leaves.
2. Add one pinch of your homemade chai masala powder.
3. Add milk and sugar and let it boil.
4. Sieve the tea using a strainer.
5. Savour and enjoy!

I love this refreshing and naturally aromatic tea. The best part is how light it is, that it doesn't leave your stomach feeling loaded, and it also has loads of health benefits. The cardamom is an antioxidant and has a mild, sweet taste. Pepper is anti-inflammatory and great for digestion. Dry ginger improves immunity and is particularly helpful to fight coughs and colds during seasonal weather changes. Cinnamon sticks add a unique, sweet taste and warmth to the tea and help regulate sugar consumption. Cloves are particularly helpful in relieving expecting mothers' aches and pains and helping in the baby's brain development. Nutmeg regulates heart and liver functioning. Tulsi leaves, often called Holy Basil, have immense benefits such as warding off infections, regulating your blood pressure, and keeping pregnancy-induced nausea at bay. Saffron, because of its 'cold' nature, is one of the most potent and natural mood up-lifters. It helps cure morning sickness and greatly aides in improving digestion.

When it comes to snacking options, I cut out unnecessary items like fried food, processed food, maida, refined sugars, and even reduced my intake of salt and spices. I kept my fridge well-stocked with fresh, seasonal fruits, to snack on in between meals. Along with providing much-needed vitamins, fruits also help satisfy your palate. As with vegetables, it is best to stick to local varieties with fruits as well, as they give you the freshest options. Nuts are another healthy go-to option. I would soak ten almonds overnight and have them in the morning. I also made my own trail mix with dried fruits and nuts to carry on the go. Walnuts, dates, figs, and chilgoza (pine nuts) are popular options, but you can include pretty much any seed or nut you prefer.

I have a taste for savoury food, so I came up with some innovative snack ideas to munch on. Raw or sautéed paneer with a dash of roasted cumin powder and black salt masala is a personal favourite. I frequently had red quinoa salad with broccoli and bell peppers too. Meat eaters can make this even more filling by adding steamed chicken. All of these snacks are rich in protein, which helps in building and repairing the tissues in your body. Homemade bhelpuri and murmurey with puffed rice, and a side of mint and tamarind chutney, is, of course, a classic in Indian households. It is

Enjoying Every Morsel: A Wholesome and Healthy Diet

low on calories while satisfying our craving for tanginess.

Potatoes are a desi staple and can be enjoyed in many different forms. I particularly enjoy boiled or roasted potatoes. These are filling without being heavy. I enjoyed this dish for dinner because it saved me from the uninvited yet regular problem of heartburn and acid regurgitation. My tummy felt light, and my heart was happy.

MAKING DELICIOUS AND HEALTHY POTATO DISH

Ingredients required for 2 servings:

1. Large sized potatoes – 2 to 3 pieces
2. Crushed roasted peanuts – 2 tablespoons
3. Chopped green chilies – 2 in nos.
4. Chopped coriander leaves – 1 tablespoon
5. Cumin seeds – 1 teaspoon
6. Ghee – 2 teaspoons
7. Crushed black pepper (not powdered) – ¼ teaspoon
8. Salt – ½ teaspoon

Method of preparation:

1. Wash and clean the potatoes well.
2. Put them in a pressure cooker. Add 2 cups of water and 1/2 teaspoon of salt.
3. Cook the potatoes for 25 minutes on a low fire.

4. Once the pressure releases on its own, open the pressure cooker. Discard the excess water.
5. Peel the potatoes when they are slightly warm, and lightly mash them with a fork.
6. Add the freshly chopped green chilies, chopped coriander, crushed peanuts, and crushed pepper to the coarsely mashed potato.
7. Take a pan and heat it. Add ghee, and when it becomes smoky, add the cumin seeds until they pop. Garnish the potato mix with this seasoning.
8. Your sumptuous snack is ready. Relish it!

For those with a sweet tooth, a sugar craving can be so intense that it can drive you to tears. It feels like nothing can fully satisfy the pining besides jalebis and laddoos dripping with dalda. But these are precisely the forms of sugar that you should be avoiding. I gave sweet fruits a go and when this did not completely appease my sugar pang, I discovered a healthier and more satisfying option. I simply added them to a bowl of curd with jaggery granules or crushed jaggery. Curd is easy on the stomach, since it aids digestion and cools the body down. The combination is also rich in iron and calcium, both of which are vital during pregnancy.

A word to the wise: do not cut out ghee from your diet. Previously considered highly fattening, it has now been proven by research to have many valuable effects on the

Enjoying Every Morsel: A Wholesome and Healthy Diet

body that cannot be substituted by anything else. Ghee is rich in omega-3 fatty acids that maintain heart and brain health. It boosts the immune system and helps with digestion. So, have your ghee with rice, roti or dal, and remember to enjoy and cherish its impact on your life and the life of your child. Unlike in my first pregnancy, I made a conscious effort to have ghee regularly during my second one and enjoyed its benefits in terms of improved stamina and higher energy levels.

I must point out that I managed to sustain a healthy diet because I also made provisions for 'cheat days'. These were days when I allowed myself to indulge in the non-healthy, delicious food that I had been consciously cutting out of my life. One day a week, I gave myself a free pass to have fries, pasta, and samosas. But here again, I made sure to restrain myself from going overboard; I told myself that this was not the last time I would be savouring these delicacies. The cheat day would come again the next week. And it would be truly enjoyable only if I had eaten healthy the rest of the week. After all, I had made a conscious commitment to myself and my child. As always, I was a staunch believer in myself, and that was how I could sail through.

3

AVERTING THE EVIDENCE: KEEPING STRETCH MARKS AT BAY

When you think of a pregnant woman, the first image that might pop into your mind is that of an enlarged belly. That is the most telltale sign of pregnancy. There is something very pure and beautiful about pregnancy, about a mother on the verge of bringing new life into this earth. Both the times I was pregnant, I found myself pondering over the sheer perfection of the human body, particularly the female body. I was awash in humility and tinged with pride at having been chosen by Nature to be the bearer of this sacred ability.

For most women, a pregnant stomach isn't big and

Averting the Evidence: Keeping Stretch Marks at Bay

round from the get-go. In fact, the bump starts to be noticeable only from the second trimester. This is when all the congratulations from one and all start to pour in. As your belly grows, the skin on your body stretches rapidly to accommodate the baby. More often than not, though, the stomach is not the only area that bears signs of this change. Your arms, your back, your thighs and legs are just as susceptible to stretch marks.

Stretch marks could also be the reason that you stop wearing your favourite sarees and sleeveless dresses. They will stay as evidence of the battle that your body went through in bringing your child to this earth. There are many who will tell you that these are marks of beauty—and so they can be, depending on your own taste! When it came to me, I found no beauty in my stretch marks. As a habitually fit and toned person, I wanted to overcome this natural but avoidable outcome of pregnancy.

My mother had warned me that stretch marks are some of the most stubborn skin issues that a woman faces. Once they set in, they are practically impossible to get rid of. Even complex and extremely expensive laser treatments are often not good enough. The only effective measure to handle stretch marks is to prevent them from appearing in the first place. I thought of it as a race against time, with weight gain and the serpentine marks it leaves on the body as my opponents, and I wanted to win by a wide margin!

Grow Your Baby, Not Your Weight

Even though weight gain *will certainly* be a part of your pregnancy, it does not have to be sudden or immense. All expecting mothers need to constantly keep in mind that they are in complete control of their own fitness. It will require patience and commitment, but it is entirely possible to stay fit during this process. The secret to preventing abrupt changes in weight is by sticking to the right food and reasonable portion sizes. Daily moderate exercise is also non-negotiable. Tripling your portion sizes might seem like a good way to manage the whirlwind pregnancy emotions, but the resulting weight gain will cause you grief in the long run. On the other hand, a slow and sustained routine of good eating habits will keep you feeling your absolute best.

Looking back, I am proud of achieving my goal of preventing stretch marks from appearing on my body. I take great satisfaction in it, especially since I did not need the help of fancy skin treatments and legions of skin experts constantly monitoring me. I want to emphasise this, because it is something that everyone has the potential to achieve.

Of course, I *did* have one expert with me every step of the way: my wonderful mother. My mother was actually the one who brought to my attention that I could take care of my stretch marks. She insisted that I focus on skin care with as much seriousness and consistency as I invested in my medical needs, right from the first trimester.

The first step is understanding why stretch marks occur

Averting the Evidence: Keeping Stretch Marks at Bay

in the first place. The reason is simple: your belly expands at a very quick pace, physiologically speaking, and the epidermal layer has to keep up with this speed. As the skin expands quickly, the collagen and elastin compounds that support the skin tend to rupture, leaving a band-like scarring. When women end up gaining weight all over their bodies while expecting and not just on their belly, the same process of rapid stretching occurs in other parts of the body as well.

An irritating side effect of the growing belly and stretch marks is itching. For some lucky women, the itching remains mild. For most expecting mothers, though, itching is a persistent occurrence that begins in the fourth or fifth month and increases progressively. Just like with acne and chicken pox, the worst thing you can possibly do is to give in to the sensation and scratch. Since it is a definite route to scarring, I did everything to avoid itching at all costs.

> **Dr Rekha on itching and other complications arising during pregnancy:** Intrahepatic Cholestasis of Pregnancy (IHCP), Gestational Diabetes Mellitus, Eclampsia arising from hypertension, and low lying placenta or placenta previa are not common problems and would need requisite medical care corresponding with diagnosis. These conditions have symptoms such as itching all over the body, headaches, blurring of vision, bleeding, etc. and require immediate medical attention.

Grow Your Baby, Not Your Weight

More difficult than while awake, I needed to prevent scratching myself in my sleep too. Until this became a habit, I wore soft socks on my hands when going to bed, to keep the nails at bay!

I realized that the most crucial step in managing itchiness and stretch marks is moisturising. Rapidly expanding skin tends to dry out easily, which exacerbates both the marks and the itchiness. It is, in fact, a vicious circle of dryness and itchiness feeding into each other, with stretch marks as the final outcome. I made it a point to moisturise my belly at least twice a day, without fail. I made it a part of my daily ritual after my bath, in the morning, and before turning in for the night. I have noticed that we tend to make excuses to avoid doing things that are good for us, beginning with the all-time favourite, 'I don't have enough time.' However, I found that it takes an average of thirty seconds to massage some lotion on your stomach—I timed myself over a week to get an estimate. Surely, you can spend an extra thirty seconds, twice a day, for yourself!

Any good quality moisturiser is a safe bet. You do not need fancy products from luxury brands that promise immediate transformation—that is simply a marketing gimmick. I, for one, went the homemade route. My mother is a magician, the king and queen of creams and body care. When she told me about stretch marks, she shared her secret recipe for a moisturising cream that women in her

Averting the Evidence: Keeping Stretch Marks at Bay

family have used for generations, with impeccable results. It is surprisingly easy to make, and once made, it lasts for a good 3 to 4 months.

MOM'S MAGIC CREAM TO PREVENT STRETCH MARKS

Ingredients:
1. Pure Shea butter - 100 g
2. Any cold cream as a base - 250 g
3. Vaseline petroleum jelly - 10 g
4. Cold-pressed virgin coconut oil or olive oil - 10 ml
5. Almond oil - 10 ml
6. Lavender essential oil - 10 drops

Method of preparation:
1. Take a vessel with boiling hot water and keep another vessel containing shea butter in it so that it melts under the heat. Do not heat the shea butter directly or let the water enter it.
2. Remove the vessel of shea butter and mix all the ingredients together until it has a uniform consistency. Use a blender if necessary.
3. Store it in an airtight container.
4. Use the smooth, fragrant cream all over your body, especially on your belly, twice a day, after bathing and before going to bed.

Grow Your Baby, Not Your Weight

The 'magic' cream prevents dryness, soothes itchy skin, and keeps the skin lubricated, with elasticity intact. It also makes the skin soft and supple.

Another useful tip from my mother's repertoire was to apply muslin cloths to soothe the itching. The feel of the soft cloth reduces skin irritation. Applying a wet towel on the belly area also has a soothing effect, with the added bonus of helping reduce acidity and bloating. When you are pregnant, it is a good time to invest in an aloe vera plant for your home. No store-bought gel will be as pure, and therefore as effective, as the fresh sap that you can extract from your plant's leaves. This is an excellent choice of lotion to apply on your stretched skin. Homemade neem packs, made by grinding soaked neem leaves and mixing them with honey and yogurt in equal parts, also do wonders for the skin. Moreover, neem's antibacterial properties help stave off possible infections.

Indian weather conditions are such that we have to constantly deal with extremes. It is either scorching hot or freezing cold. Thus, it is hardly surprising that these extremes have a damaging impact on the skin, along with other parts of the body. During pregnancy, you must pamper your body a little. Frequent baths help alleviate itching. But bath water is best kept at a lukewarm temperature. It may be tempting to use cold water for relief in summer, and piping hot baths are the ultimate luxury in winter. But the baby growing inside you needs tenderness, and so do

Averting the Evidence: Keeping Stretch Marks at Bay

you. Lukewarm water can provide that, and this moderate temperature is also ideal for keeping the skin hydrated. Unlike extreme temperatures, lukewarm water will not dry out the skin. Remember to use a mild soap, and you're all set for a happy bath.

Another tip that should come as no surprise, but far too often does, is that stretching exercises help prevent stretch marks. Exercising keeps you fit and flexible, and when the body is familiar with the sensation of stretching, through different poses, the skin becomes attuned to it. This reduces collagen rupture and allows the skin to expand without leaving marks. There were a few exercises that I swore by during my pregnancy. However, these should be performed only after consulting your gynaecologist, and in the presence of expert guidance.

The following pictures illustrate these stretching exercises. They are simple to perform and evoke tremendous confidence and amazement at one's own stretchability thresholds. Hold each posture for a minimum of 10 seconds and progressively increase it to 20 seconds as your capacity increases. Then, repeat on the other side. You can easily perform each exercise a minimum of 3 times.

Enjoy your stretching, your balancing act, and the indescribable feeling it gives you!

Remember to enjoy the view of the sky, too, the clouds, and the one and only Sun!

Grow Your Baby, Not Your Weight

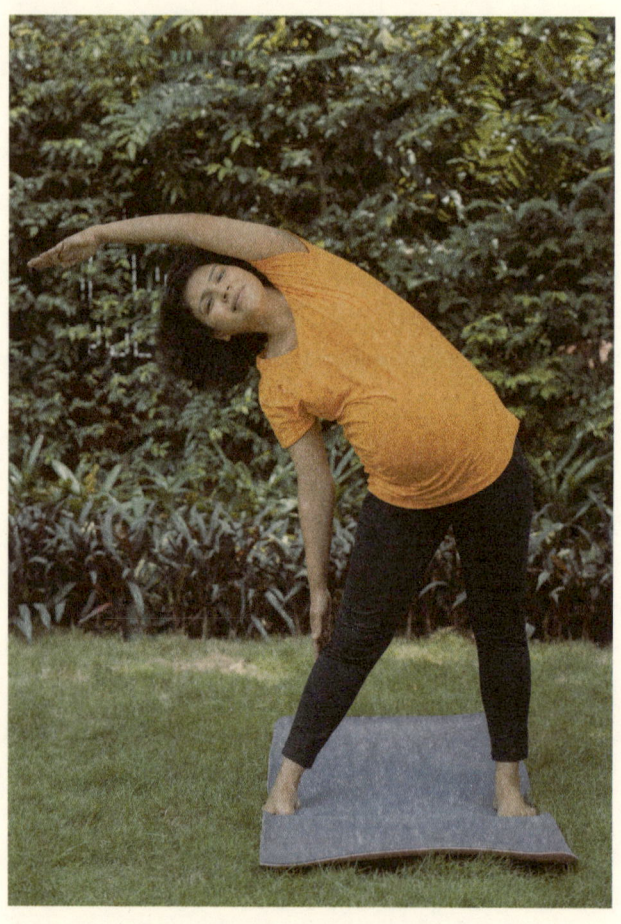

1: Open your legs as wide as the distance between your shoulders. Bend your right shoulder, your right hand reaching out to your right knee. Bend a little more and stretch out your left arm horizontally over your head towards your right side. A trick here is to touch your left upper arm to your left ear. Make sure you keep both your knees straight. Repeat the same for the right side.

Averting the Evidence: Keeping Stretch Marks at Bay

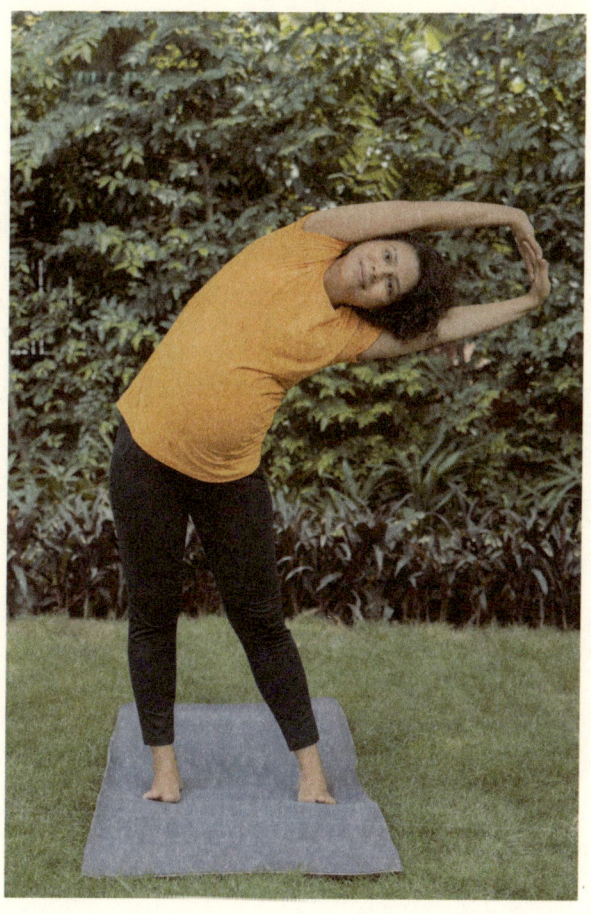

2: Again, open your legs as wide as the distance between your shoulders. Stretch out your arms and hold the palms outwards towards the sky in an interlocked position. Now, gently bend towards the left side with the entire left side of your body stretching. Your arms should be absolutely straight and stretched out, touching your ears. Repeat the same for the right side.

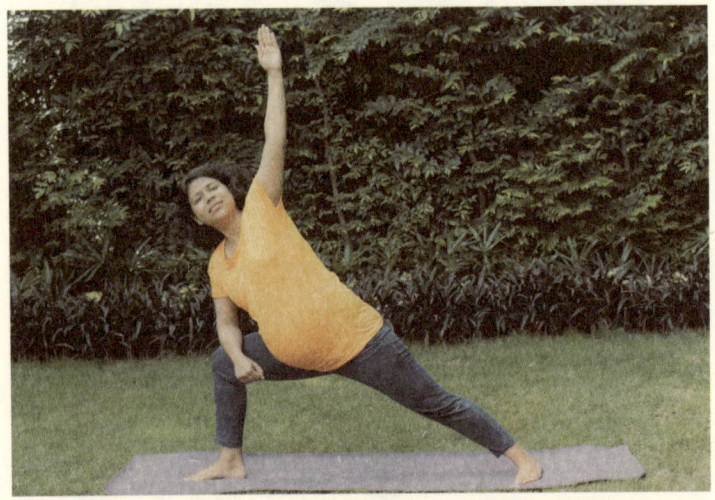

3: Stretch your legs as you stand. Move your right foot towards the right side, bend your right knee and gently place your right forearm on your bent right knee. Now, gradually lift your left arm upwards and make sure you keep it straight. Imagine that you are being pulled upwards. Ensure that your left knee doesn't bend. Repeat the same for the right side.

Averting the Evidence: Keeping Stretch Marks at Bay

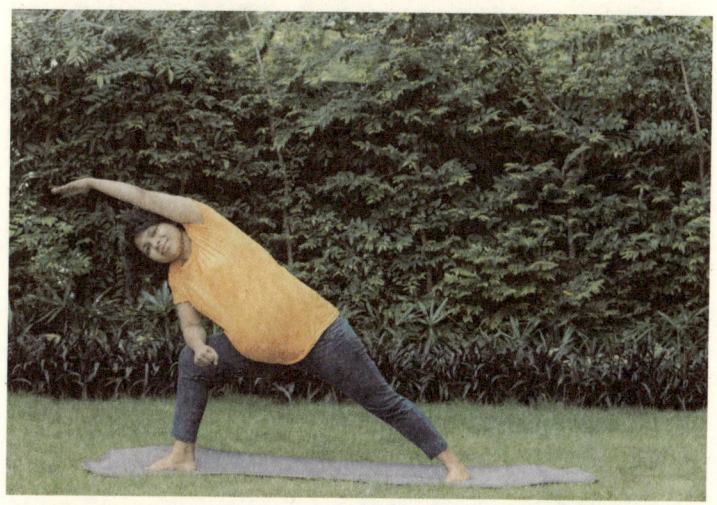

4: Again, stretch your legs as you stand. Move your right foot towards the right side, bend your right knee and gently place your right forearm on your bent right knee. Now, gradually lift your left arm horizontally over your head towards the right side and make sure you keep it straight, touching your left ear with your left upper arm. Ensure that your left knee doesn't bend. Feel the stretch of the entire left side of your body. Repeat the same for the right side.

Grow Your Baby, Not Your Weight

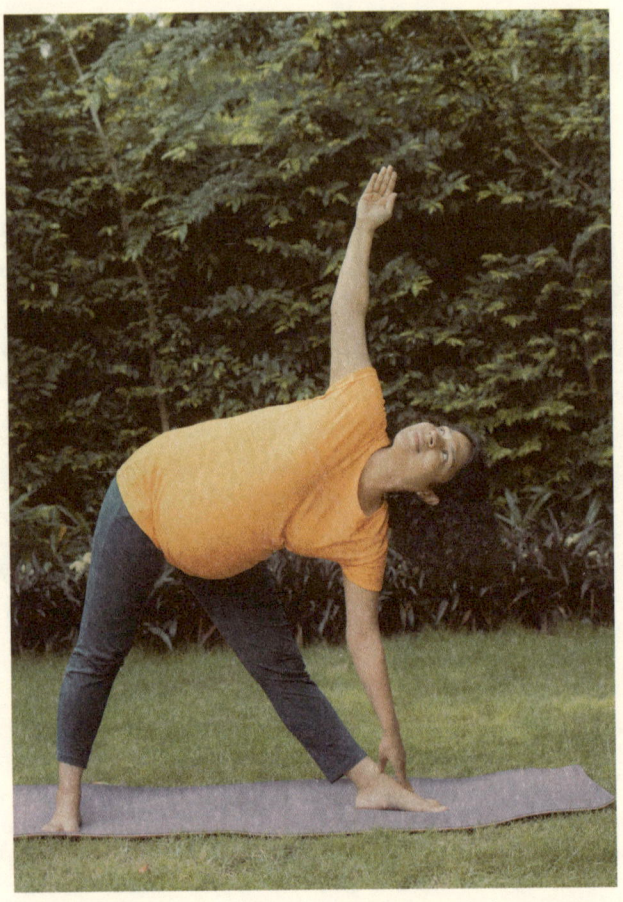

5: Trikonasana: Stretch your legs as you stand. Open your left foot towards the right side and gently place your fingers from your left hand onto your left foot. Now, gradually lift your right arm upwards and make sure you keep it straight. Both your arms should be aligned in a single line. Ensure that your knees don't bend. Repeat the same for the left side.

Averting the Evidence: Keeping Stretch Marks at Bay

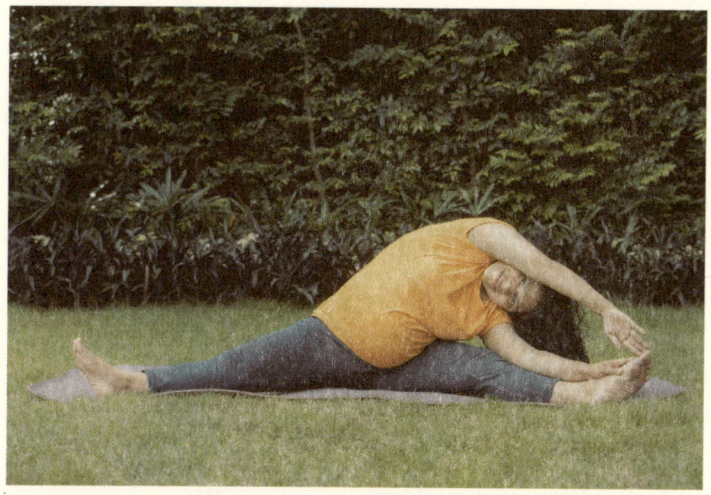

6: Sit down and stretch your legs out as wide as you can. Lift up your arms and move your entire upper body along with your arms to your left side. Try to touch your left foot with both your hands. Ensure you don't bend your knees. Repeat the same for the left side.

A pregnant woman is a powerhouse. Something as insignificant as an irritating itch cannot be allowed to bother her unduly. I treated this phase as an opportunity to discover new ways of self-care and pampering, which ultimately led to a healthier body and a happier mind. Just remember to start your care and management early. After all, a bit of extra loving can never go to waste!

4

SPARKLE FROM WITHIN: GLOWING SKIN

During the European Renaissance, there emerged a belief that internal beauty and purity were reflected on the outside—that a person with a beautiful soul could not help but be just as pleasant to look at. Of course, that is not how science works, but what we do know is that what we put into our bodies has an impact on our external appearances. From our skin to our hair, nails, and teeth, everything is closely and intimately linked to the internal processes and functions of our bodies and minds. Thus, a well-maintained interior invariably leads to an appealing exterior.

Sparkle from Within: Glowing Skin

Pregnancy creates a veritable hormonal whirlpool in our bodies. Within a few short months, the quantity of hormones—particularly oestrogen and progesterone—being produced in the body increases dramatically. These hormonal changes prepare the body to host the new baby, but far too often, they wreak havoc on the poor mother's own system. They cause frequent and unpredictable mood swings, exhaustion, nausea, and digestive issues, even heartburn. As if all of this was not enough, pesky skin issues often crop up as a result of hormonal imbalances.

The significant increase in the blood flow within the body gives some fortunate women a glow from within, or the 'pregnancy glow'. For most of us, though, pimples and dull skin are the norm. Some even suffer from another kind of pregnancy marker on the face, the 'pregnancy mask' or melasma that takes place because of hyper pigmentation. Our diets have a very important role to play in this. As we have discussed in the previous chapters, we need to be very conscious of our dietary habits during this period. Pregnant women's faces can become puffy or swell up, making her look and feel underconfident or unlike herself.

We have often heard talk about putting our 'best foot forward' in important scenarios, meaning it is important to make a good impression. Thus, we need to make sure that our faces tell a compelling story about our personalities.

In Indian families, some of us would have heard from

relatives that it is a good sign for a woman to have a plump and round face, as it indicates that she comes from a well-to-do family that takes care of its daughters. However, I prefer a lean, smooth face, where your cheek bones and nose look sharper. This is much easier to achieve than most women think, even during pregnancy. Like almost every other tip in this book, this requires patience, consistency, and persistence. So, let's keep the chubby cheeked roundness for the baby in the belly, and focus on acquiring smooth skin on a toned face that can then do all the talking for us!

Weight gained on one's face is the first to make an appearance, and the last to leave, if it ever does. In fact, it is extremely difficult to lose accumulated weight on the face, because the sort of rigorous exercise that leads to melting of fat is quite difficult to perform on one's face. Prevention of weight gain is really the best route to take.

First, it is important to get the basics right. The one non-negotiable aspect of your skincare routine should be water. Water is truly the elixir of life. It is practically impossible to overdo, and the benefits are too many to list out. During pregnancy, it is best to drink at least twelve glasses of water a day. Some people advise drinking it in short, frequent sips. I, for one, could not do that. I am a perpetually thirsty person, and I chug on water as an empty tank chugs on fuel. If you are like me, then you are in luck. If, on the other hand, you find yourself frequently dehydrated because

Sparkle from Within: Glowing Skin

of how little water you drink, now is the time to change that habit. Keeping a glass filled with water next to you helps. This encourages more intake than a bottle, which often goes unnoticed for hours. Make it a big tumbler. In fact, make hydration a fun game for yourself. Maybe you can time your sips and give yourself a treat when you finish a certain number, or maybe buying pretty cups and glasses will encourage you to drink water more frequently. Be as creative as you can.

Believe it or not, as a teetotaller there have been times when I felt mildly intoxicated just from drinking water! What a lovely feeling it is, enjoying the feeling of tipsiness without a drop of the damaging liquor in the body.

Water helps with another annoying pregnancy guest: pimples. Along with some H2O, a well-curated skincare routine becomes immensely important. You need to become more consistent than ever with your cleaning and moisturising routine. It is imperative that you wash your face with a mild, preferably herbal, or a chemical free face wash, every morning and evening, and follow it up with a good moisturiser. Avoiding sugar and overly oily food will also help keep pimples at bay. I used a homemade pack as a scrub once a week, which kept my pimple breakouts under reasonable control. It has the most widely available, simple ingredients and requires a maximum of 15 minutes per week to apply.

MY HOME-MADE ATTA/WHEAT FLOUR PACK

Ingredients:
1. Atta/Wheat flour – 1 tablespoon
2. Besan/Gram flour – 1/2 teaspoon
3. Curd – 1 teaspoon
4. Honey – 1/2 teaspoon
5. Lemon – 3 to 4 drops

Using the pack:
1. Clean your face with a gentle face wash
2. Mix all the ingredients in a small vessel
3. Apply this mixture on your entire face
4. Let it dry for 10-12 minutes
5. Wash your face with water
6. Apply your face moisturizer

We, Indians, with our deliciously brown skin, somehow function under the misconception that we do not need to use sunscreen. We could not be more mistaken. Sunscreen is used to protect the skin from sun damage and ultra-violet rays and has little or no connection to skin colouration. During pregnancy, when the sensitivity and chances of hyper-pigmentation of our skin are already higher than usual, sunscreen usage becomes even more important. And the SPF value of the sunscreen you use is always important. Any value below SPF 30 will not work at all, and ideally, it

Sparkle from Within: Glowing Skin

is best to choose an SPF of 50 and above. As with washing and moisturising your face, make sunscreen application a part of your morning skincare ritual. A generous dollop of sunscreen, about a teaspoon full, slathered over the face, and you are protected. Don't forget to apply it on your neck too!

Doesn't a good massage help you feel rejuvenated? Why not make it part of your facial skincare regimen? Give yourself a quick ten-minute massage once or twice a week, or as frequently as you wish to. If you are feeling more adventurous, you might want to give facial yoga a try. Massages help keep the blood flowing and the skin taut and toned. The glorious feeling of comfort it brings is an added bonus.

On to potentially less exciting options: I'm afraid that you will have to regularly work out your facial muscles to keep the weight gain on your face under control. This might not be your favourite thing to do, but the benefits are enormous. These exercises are sure to get you a swanlike neck and a jaw line that can cut cakes. So, make your face compete with your body as it works overtime, so that both are fit and fantastic by the end of it.

I have been a fitness freak all my life. I always enjoyed sports and workouts, even as a young child. When I grew older and joined the workforce, many people told me that the punishing workload might not leave me with any time or energy to continue with my exercise schedule. But something I realised over time is that people make time for whatever they prioritise. The most common 'I don't have time' problem can be easily dealt with by setting small time targets of, say, fifteen minutes a day and gradually increasing them as you start enjoying the routine. It did not take me too long to realise that I would only be able to make time for my workout in the mornings. So, I became *that* person who makes it a point to wake up at six in the morning to complete their workout routine before getting ready for the day.

Despite such a vigorous lifestyle, though, I have a naturally roundish face, which didn't match up with the tautness of my body after I exercised. But the special care I took during pregnancy changed this. It turns out that spot weight reduction does work, at least for the face, if only one can figure out the right exercise routine for it. I was delighted that these exercises helped me to finally get rid of the extra facial flab and get the toned look I had always wanted. My husband Abhishek was amazed and true to his large heartedness, he was and continues to be full of compliments.

I was very lucky to find an extremely dedicated and modest yoga trainer, Ms Sushila Biswas, who made my face exercises a strict and indispensable part of my everyday pre-natal yoga routine. With profound gratitude to her, I share some very helpful facial exercises. These exercises brought me closer to my desired goal—the Nefertiti look I had grown up seeing in school textbooks and had always aspired towards.

Kapol Shakti Vikasak Kriya: Kapol means cheek, Shakti Vikasak means strengthening and Kriya means exercise. These exercises are akin to blowing a shankh (shell) wherein all the power of the face and mouth is used, and facial muscles are put to work. You can start doing the three exercises explained below, 5 times each, and later, a maximum of 10 times each.

First exercise:
1. Inflate your cheeks by sucking air through your mouth and hold it for 10 seconds.
2. Hold your fist to your mouth, touching your lips.
3. Blow the air out through your lips, very slowly, into the hole in your fist.
4. Make sure you feel the pressure on your entire cheeks as you blow the air out.

Second exercise:
1. Open your palms and join the fingers of both your palms with each other.
2. Place your left thumb on left nostril and right thumb on right nostril keeping your elbows in a straight line.

3. Open your mouth and take in as much air as possible.
4. Lower your face so that your little fingers touch your chest.
5. Hold your breath for ten seconds and then gently release the air through your nose.

Third exercise:
1. Inflate your cheeks by sucking air through your mouth.
2. Place one of your index fingers on your lips, sealing them.
3. Hold this for 10 seconds.
4. Gently release the air through your nose.

Exercise for double chin:
1. Move your neck backwards as much as you can.
2. Open your jaw as much as you can and close. Repeat 20 to 30 times.
3. Move your neck back to its normal position.
4. Repeat the above steps 2 to 3 times.

With a sense of pride, I can now say that a naturally contoured, toned, and glowing face is possible during pregnancy. In fact, pregnancy is as good a time as any to strive for it, have it, and enjoy it for the rest of your life.

5

WEIGHT IN CHECK: YOGA AND WALKING

As someone who has stayed lean her entire life, I worried about becoming several sizes bigger during pregnancy. My fears were heightened by all the unwanted sympathy I started receiving from women around me. 'Oh, its normal to get out of shape during pregnancy,' or 'Now that you are expecting, be ready to throw out all of your favourite clothes and get a new wardrobe several sizes bigger. You will never fit into your old clothes again.' But I was not about to be swayed by what people around me had to say. As always, I believed in following my doctor's advice and my own gut feelings about my body. My doctor reassured me that I would not necessarily put on too much

Grow Your Baby, Not Your Weight

weight, as long as I was careful and systematic with my diet and exercise routine. The baby in me needed to grow, not myself!

What we often refuse to acknowledge is that excessive body weight is not merely an aesthetic issue. In fact, external appearance would ideally only play a small role in the entire debate. Gaining weight has many unfortunate side effects on one's level of health and fitness. Everyday activities become more difficult to perform, and one has to deal with a variety of lifestyle-related health issues such as diabetes and hypertension. Obesity has also been proved to have exacerbating effects on other deadly diseases, including certain forms of cancer.

During pregnancy, too, it is very important to keep one's weight in check. Pregnancy is a time when the mother's health becomes her top priority, because it is her duty to keep her baby healthy as well. If the mother experiences a lowered state of health, this will invariably impact the overall nourishment of the child. Pregnancy weight gain has the unfortunate side effect of causing gestational diabetes in some women. This is a form of diabetes that occurs specifically during pregnancy due to high levels of blood sugar in the expecting mother. It is usually detected towards the end of the second trimester of pregnancy. Gestational diabetes occurs due to several reasons, including hormonal imbalance. This form of diabetes is temporary, though, and

Weight in Check: Yoga and Walking

the mother can definitely keep it under control by watching her diet and exercising.

> **Dr Rekha on exercise during pregnancy:** It is recommended that a mother-to-be maintains some amount of low to moderate physical exercise throughout her pregnancy. For those who already maintain a regular workout routine, it may be possible to continue moderate intensity workouts such as aerobics. For others, low impact workout routines such as walking, stretching, and yoga can be practiced. Any form of strenuous exercise that can cause injury or risk of fall should be strictly avoided. Excess fatigue can have adverse effects on both mother and child. In cases in which the expecting mother has certain underlying conditions such as heart diseases, hypertension or intrauterine growth restriction of the baby (IUGR), a sedentary lifestyle may be medically advised.

During my pregnancy, I decided to focus on my physical health by preparing a detailed workout regimen for myself, right from the early days. I planned to work out at least five days a week, for forty-five minutes to an hour. Some might find this too stringent, given that exhaustion levels are already high for the woman during pregnancy. However, I had the advantage of being an active person already. A regular exercise routine had been an integral part of my life for a long time, so this was not a new or significantly different inclusion in my daily routine. My body, too, was used to a fair deal of physical exertion, so I did not have to worry about injuring myself by trying to inculcate some new forms of pregnancy-specific exercises. It is important that your own routine is comfortable and that you enjoy it. Listen to your body and steer clear of overdoing it or overexerting under all circumstances!

Another reason why I made a tough schedule for myself was that I realised that only rigorous discipline would help me meet my target of staying fit and flab-free. Inconsistent exercising does not have a very high impact on overall weight loss. So, exercising just a few days a week with long gaps in between would not help. In fact, I told myself that if I was ever too tired, I would rather shorten the duration of working out occasionally than skip it completely. It was not a leeway that I allowed myself too often, usually pushing for forty-five minutes of exercise. Admittedly, some days were much more difficult than others. On those days, I told myself that it was okay to relax and just let go.

The easiest form of working out that anyone can do, in one manner or the other, is walking. Unlike most other forms of exercise, walking continues to be a safe option at every stage of pregnancy, with no risks to the mother or the baby. We have already talked about my love affair with morning walks in the fresh air, and how they helped me bring

Weight in Check: Yoga and Walking

morning sickness and nausea under control. You could go out for walks on the road or at a park, early in the morning, in the evening, or late at night. The time of day and duration can be adjusted based on factors such as location, safety issues, and convenience. For those lucky enough to live close to nature—by the beach, in the mountains, or even near a forested area, a walk can also be an opportunity to enjoy the beauty of nature. If the English got one thing right in the Victorian era, it was their love for long walks, at every hour of the day. And if you can get a friend or family member to come along, this is also a fantastic way to bond with them. If walking outside is impossible, just walk around your terrace or even your own house! There can be no excuse for not walking, except the lack of initiative and willpower.

Once you enter your second trimester of pregnancy, it is time to create a more varied exercise routine—with a clear go-ahead from your doctor, of course! The second trimester is often termed the 'golden trimester'. This is when your body has settled into its state of pregnancy. The baby has grown into a stable little foetus. Your morning sickness has possibly subsided, making your life significantly less miserable, and allowing you to enjoy your meals once again, without being afraid of throwing it all up. Now, you can be more focused on maintaining your weight and fitness. The second trimester is also the time when your body and belly start to gain weight. It therefore becomes all the more important to stretch and remain supple, and to stick to the regimen that you set for yourself.

What kept me going through my workout regime was the knowledge that I was doing it for my baby as much as for myself. When the mother gains too much weight during pregnancy, it also leads to the baby being overweight at birth. Doctors recommend that a baby's ideal weight at birth should be between 2.5 and 3 kilograms. Anything over 3 kgs makes delivery more difficult. However, walking and exercises have a proportional impact on the chances of a smooth labour transition and normal delivery. I wanted to give myself a perfect pregnancy experience, as far as possible, and to me, that meant hoping for a normal delivery. I was aware that the recent popular tendency was to get a C-section, but I was of the firm opinion that following the natural process would ultimately be of greater value to me and my child. It would ease and hasten my recovery process as well, and I wanted to be up on my feet and hands-on with my baby as soon as possible.

The traditional Indian lifestyle, with vigorous, daily physical exertion for women in the family, had a conducive effect on childbirth. The frequent use of the squatting position, be it for household chores like cooking and cleaning, or for one's regular ablutions, helped keep the muscles in the pelvic region strong and flexible, facilitating normal birth with much more ease. Nowadays, although women are busier

Weight in Check: Yoga and Walking

than ever before, our work tends to be sedentary. We sit at our desks and peer at our computer screens for long hours, before coming home and crashing on the couch in front of the television. Physical mobility and flexibility have taken a backseat, and we have to pay the price for this with health issues and difficulties during childbirth. Nevertheless, being conscious about a strict exercise routine during pregnancy can surely combat a lot of these difficulties.

As an expecting mother, you have to keep an eye on ideal weight recommendations by the doctor. When you have a workout regimen drawn up, along with ideal weights at different points of the pregnancy, it is important to keep track and see how you are performing. The weight gain could creep up on you and lead to unexpected extra kilos.

I recorded my weight on a chart that I had drawn up for the nine months of both my pregnancies. To help me do so, I kept my weighing scale under my bed, so that it was the first thing I could check in the morning. This kept sudden, significant weight fluctuations in check. This information also gave me the power to plan my meals and allow myself occasional treats accordingly. My doctor had told me that based on the pre-pregnancy weight and health conditions, a woman usually gains between ten and twelve kilos of weight during gestation, without affecting her health or the baby's. I decided to spread out the weight gain over the months, as far as possible, so that I did not have to worry about sudden dietary restrictions in the later months. I knew women who had gained too much weight in the first six months and had been advised by their doctors to be more vigilant for the third semester. They had all sorts of delicious sweets and carbs cut out of their diet, putting them in a nasty catch-22 situation of increased appetite in the last trimester along with restricted food intake. I did not wish to deal with that, and so I took action in the early months.

I started doing yoga in my fourth month of pregnancy, after receiving my doctor's approval. The benefits of yoga are well known. They extend far beyond just physical fitness. My yoga practice had a marked impact on my emotional health as well, making me feel more rejuvenated, peaceful, and happy. I combined the yogic asanas with pranayama breathwork, and together they improved my life considerably. They helped soothe my skin, improved my digestion, and increased my body's flexibility. It is because of my yoga practice that I could find relief from the inevitable cramps and leg and back aches that accompany pregnancy.

The essence of these asanas lies in pulling the entire body in an elongated position, stretching skywards to the maximum, without causing any discomfort or giddiness. You can comfortably hold each position for 10 to 20 seconds, and later, up to 30 seconds. Each asana can be done twice on both sides. But always remember to gradually release the pose by first bringing your feet to a normal position and

Weight in Check: Yoga and Walking

then bringing your arms by your sides. Breathing (inhaling/exhaling) will remain normal through the asanas.

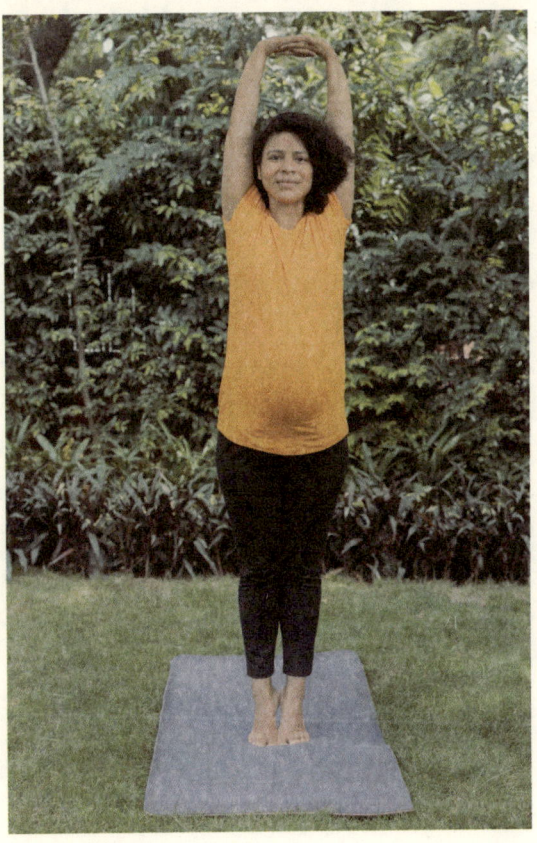

1: Tadasana: Join your feet and stand straight. Join your hands in a Namaste pose and take them upwards towards the sky. Raise your heels gently bringing your body weight onto your toes. Hold this position for 10-20 seconds, and up to 30 seconds over the next few days. You can repeat this 2 to 3 times.

Grow Your Baby, Not Your Weight

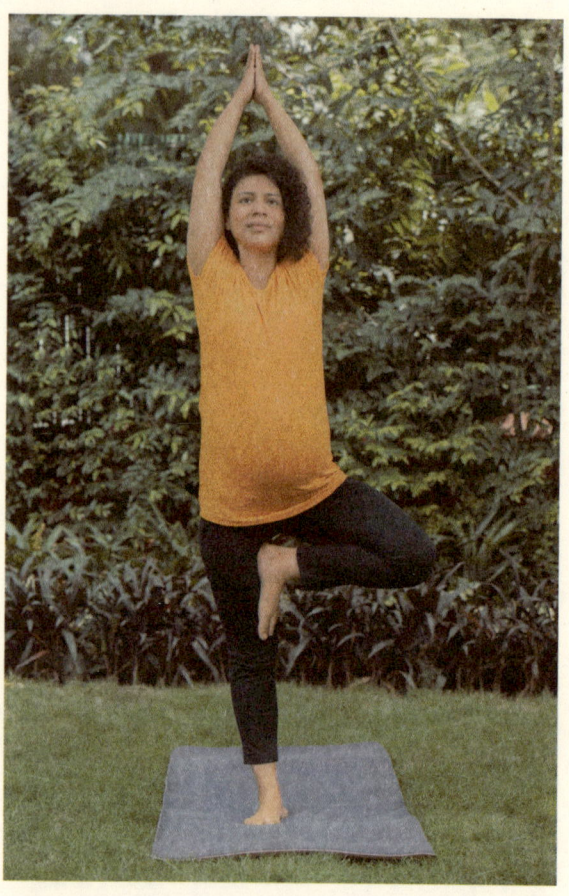

2: Vrikshasana: Join your feet and stand straight. Join your hands in a Namaste pose and take them upwards towards the sky. Raise your left foot, touching it to your right thigh. Keep the right leg and right knee straight. Hold this position. Gradually release. Repeat the other side.

Weight in Check: Yoga and Walking

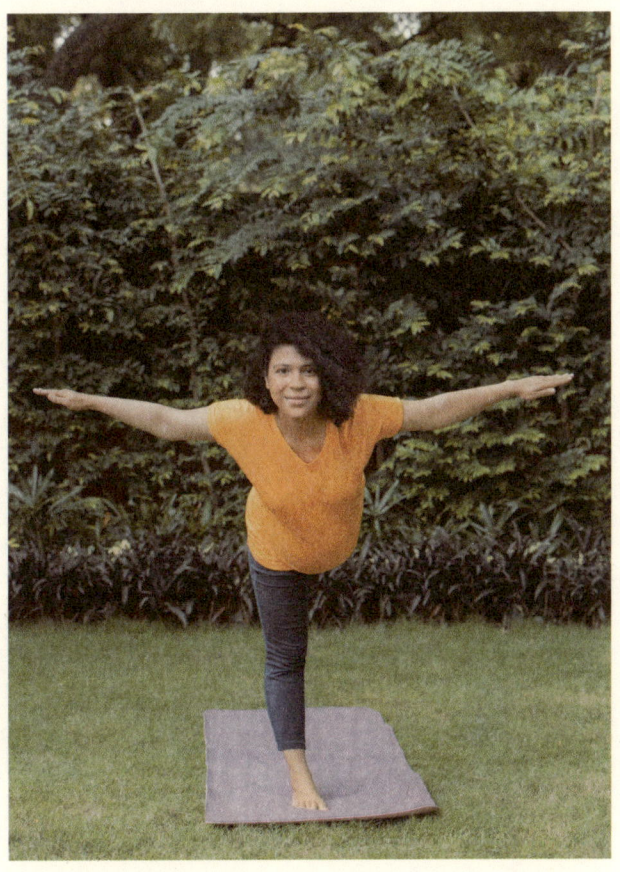

3: Warrior Pose: Join your feet and stand straight. Open your arms wide, outwards, in alignment with your shoulders. Gradually raise your left leg backwards and bend your upper body frontwards. Your right foot should take the weight of your torso and grant balance. Hold this position. Gradually release. Repeat the other side.

Grow Your Baby, Not Your Weight

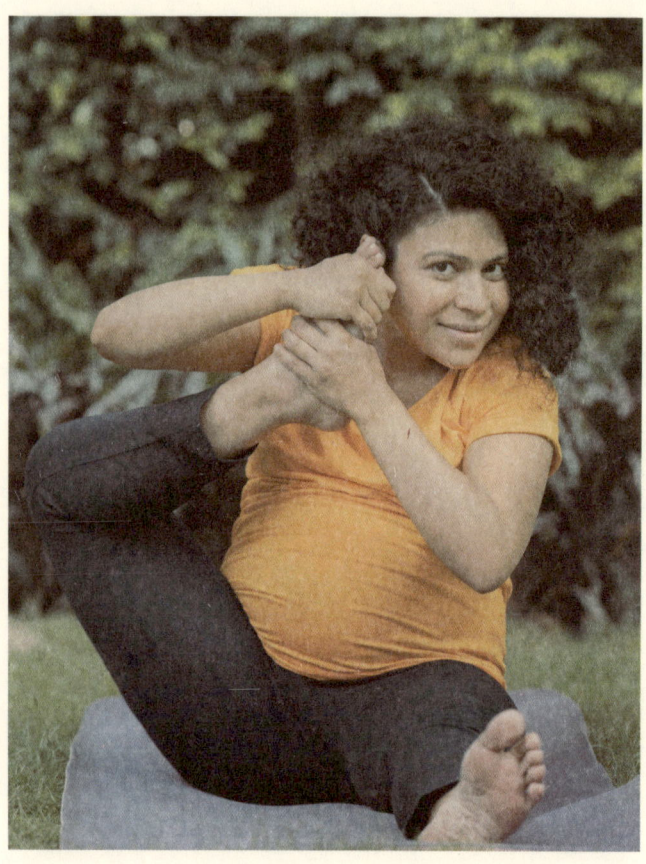

4: Akarna Dhanurasana: Sit down with your legs straight. Lift your right foot with your right hand and slowly and steadily try to take it to your right ear. Support your right foot with your left hand. Hold this position. Gradually release. Repeat the other side.

Weight in Check: Yoga and Walking

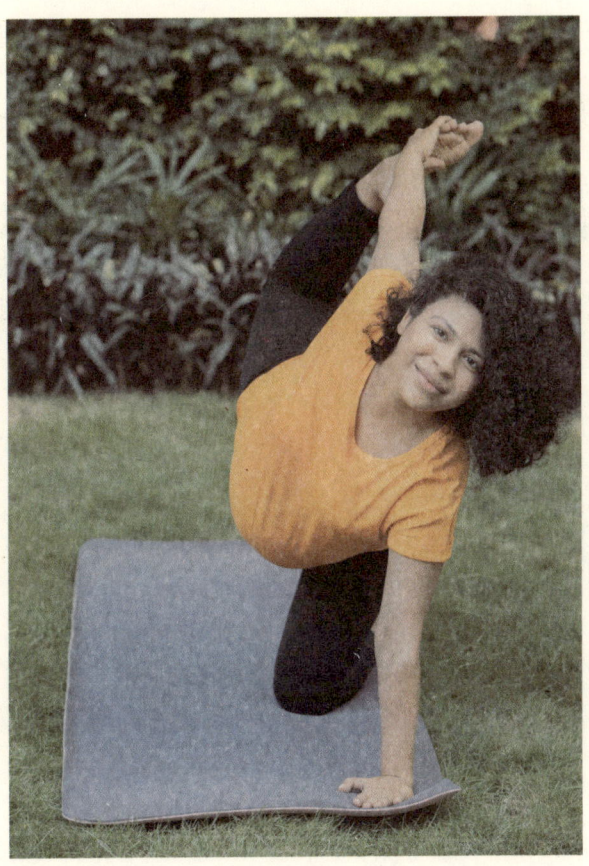

5: Tiger pose: Stand on your knees and place your left arm in front of you on the mat. Lift your right leg upwards and try to hold your right foot with your right hand, using it to further lift it upwards. Keep your left arm and left elbow straight. Hold this position. Gradually release. Repeat the other side.

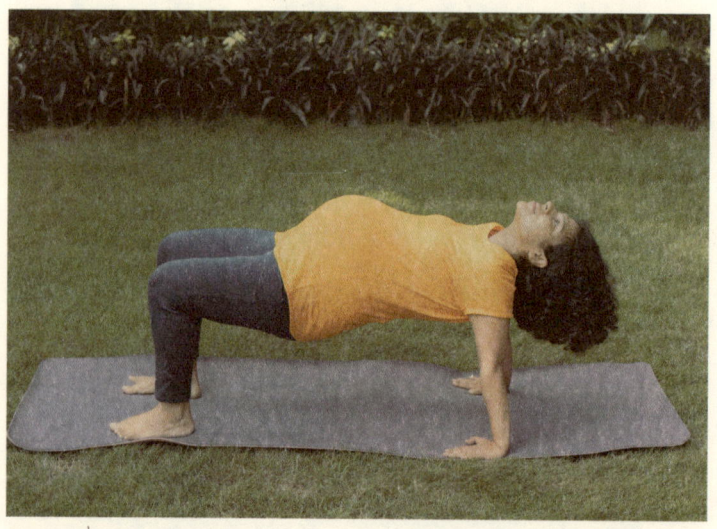

6: Ardh Chakrasana: Lie on your back with your knees folded. Place your palms on the mat and lift your body upwards. Once you are comfortable, try to straighten your back and thighs while gently pushing your belly a little outwards. Hold this position. Then, gradually release.

Weight in Check: Yoga and Walking

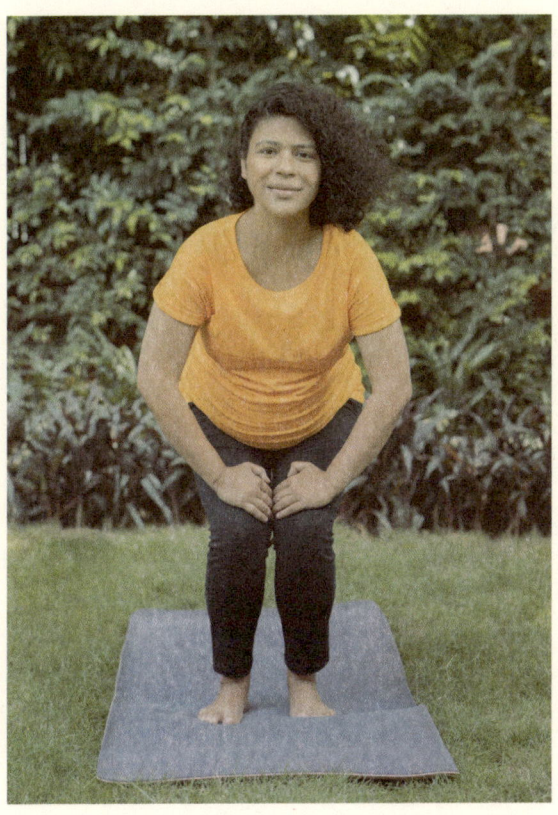

7: Knee exercises: Stand straight with a small gap between your feet. Bend your knees and hold them with your hands. Move back and forth 10 times. Next, while being in the same position, move your knees together in a clockwise direction 10 times, followed by an anti-clockwise direction 10 times. Lastly, rotate your knees together in a reverse direction i.e., the left in a clockwise and right in an anti-clockwise direction, followed by the left in an anti-clockwise and right in a clockwise direction, 10 times each.

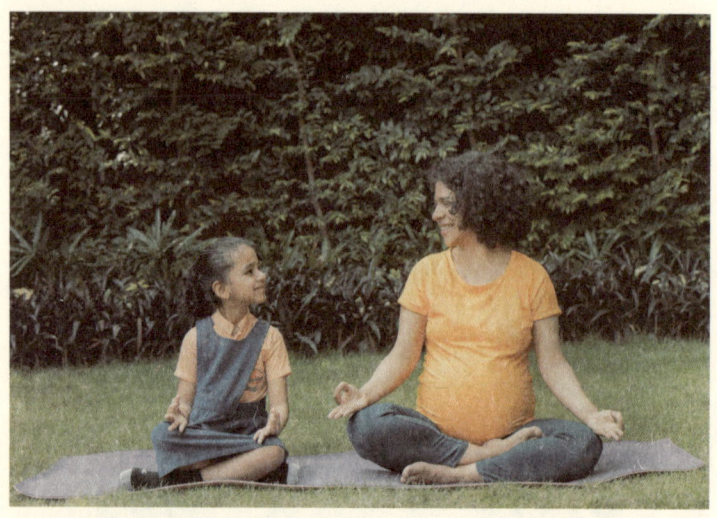

8: With my 6-year-old daughter Dania. We draw mutual admiration and inspiration from each other!

Following these rules and practices, I gained just about eight and nine kilos respectively during both my pregnancies. My babies were born at healthy weights of 2.75 kilos and 2.86 kilos. This entire experience made me more confident and fit than ever, and I can honestly say that I started living an even healthier life after becoming a mother! I hope that you, my dear reader, will also take the leap of faith and inculcate a consistent yoga practice in your routine. The benefits that you will derive will far outlive the pregnancy period and give you a happier, healthier life.

Having two children made me experience true bliss

Weight in Check: Yoga and Walking

in life, while also taking away any free time I ever had earlier. But I have maintained a consistent workout habit throughout my life, and I believe it is something everyone needs to maintain. As a busy career woman, I know that time often comes at a premium, but the value of even fifteen minutes of stretching a day will multiply manifold in terms of long-term health. As new mothers, we tend to have crazy schedules for tending to our little human. Sleepless nights and constant exhaustion are a given part of the process. But remember, working out is a commitment that you make for yourself, and you have to learn to honour it. Self-love is more important for a mother, perhaps, than for anybody else in the world. Unless your own cup is full, how would you look after the needs of your baby?

One of my greatest rewards has been watching my older daughter observe me while I work out, and then try out some of these poses herself. Young children learn by observing their parents, so it is your actions, more than your words, that will inculcate the right habits in them. I am sure that my children will grow up to be health conscious like their parents, and I believe that our regular commitment to working out will have a big role to play in this.

6

KEEP THAT SPINE STRAIGHT: BACK AND BULGE

When constructing a house, it is imperative that the base and pillars are strong. They support the entire weight of the house and ensure that the structure does not collapse under a little pressure. Plants have stems and trees have trunks to hold them up. Creepers, like the money plant, that do not have their own strong stem, have to be supported externally by sticks that prop them up. Without a firm, upright pillar or trunk, these mighty structures are unable to function. The human body is no different. For us, it is the backbone or spine that keeps us up and going.

Keep that Spine Straight: Back and Bulge

The spinal cord is an extension of the human brain, and the epicentre of the nervous system. Along with the brain, this is the body's control room. The spine grants the body with mobility and provides support and flexibility. Any damage to the spinal cord can be crippling.

When we are pregnant, the baby bump takes up most of our attention. Ask any expecting mother, and she will tell you that her first priority is to keep her belly area protected from any form of impact. Of course, this is natural and extremely important. But in the bid to protect our bulge, what we often forget, to our own detriment, is to take care of our backs as well. Newton officially discovered gravity when the apple fell on his head, and any woman who has given birth knows the strange feeling of being pulled towards the ground by her bump. There seems to be another, equally powerful force of horizontal gravity as well, pushing the tummy out front. Talk about double trouble!

As we move ahead in our pregnancy journey, the growing belly takes a toll on the entire body, but particularly on the back. As the size and weight of our belly increases, so does the pressure on the back to sustain this extra weight. It is almost as if the body is embroiled in a tug of war between the belly in front and the spine at the back, with each end trying to make the other one give in and bend to the pressure. This is quite a one-sided game, as the tummy has the growing baby on its side, and the poor spine does not increase in strength, allowing it to be weighed down under the new scenario. The result, of course, is that the mother has to face constant backache and stiffness, and all she can do is keep herself from lying in bed all day long!

> **Dr Rekha on backache:** Backaches are a normal part of pregnancy and occur due to the effects of the hormone progesterone, which loosens the joints in the pelvic region in preparation for labour. Squatting instead of bending while picking up things may help mitigate the pain. Backaches may be due to other causes, such as a urinary tract infection (UTI) or vaginal infections. Excessive vaginal discharge and frequent urination are common symptoms. In these cases, medical intervention and the administration of antibiotics may be necessary.

Several factors lead to backaches during pregnancy. Hormones cause the ligaments in the pelvic region to loosen in preparation for labour, causing a pain in the lower back. As the belly grows heavier, the mother's centre of gravity shifts forward. In order to prevent herself from losing balance and falling over, the mother-to-be unconsciously leans back into the spine, straining the muscles at the back. Both these are major culprits in causing aches and pains. While you cannot control the necessary hormonal changes, what you *can* do is take good care of your posture.

Keep that Spine Straight: Back and Bulge

Our modern lifestyles have made things easier and quicker for us. Technology promises the world at a touch of a button. But it takes a punishing toll on the body. Our professional lives these days revolve entirely around laptops and computers. We head to the office and park ourselves on our chairs for the next ten hours, barely getting up once or twice in between. Human bodies were not built for such a prolonged sedentary state; we were meant to move about and stay agile. Today, such biological requirements have taken a backseat.

Ironically, our 'back-seats' pay the price for this, and a pregnant woman is particularly susceptible. During pregnancy, it is imperative that we remain constantly vigilant about our posture. The most common and dangerous posture mistake that we tend to make is slouching. Think droopy shoulders and a bow shaped back. But this is not the natural state for the spine, which is supposed to look straight from ahead with a slight S-shape from the sides. The posture you keep needs to emulate this shape as far as possible. Your head and back need to be straight, with your lower back tucked inwards. Pregnancy is a good time to invest in an ergonomic chair for your office, if possible. These chairs help maintain good posture and the extra lumbar support towards the seat of the chair prevents slouching. You need to be particularly conscious of your sitting posture while at work. This is where the longest part of our days are spent, and the demands and pressures of work may keep us preoccupied. But now, more than ever, you need to focus on maintaining a good posture.

While it is important to have a good posture while sitting, this does not mean that you get to slack off at other times—while standing, walking, and even sleeping. Slouching is a dangerous habit, particularly because of how easy and comfortable it is to get into such a posture. I would scold my daughter whenever she slouched, yet somehow, I myself ended up giving in to the same temptation! This, despite being aware that we are more prone to injury from bad posture than children. Just as a child carrying a heavy school bag ends up stooping low, so does a pregnant mother with her growing belly. Both need to walk with purpose and keep their backs straight.

Have you noticed women in heels? Ever seen them slouch or hunch? A woman wearing heels has a perfect body alignment—a straight-backed stance, open shoulders, and a head held high. Moreover, it is hard to wear heels and not look extremely polished, with a dash of confidence and sophistication. If you wear heels regularly, there is no reason to give them up now. Simply switch to kitten heels, low platforms or anything your body is comfortable with. For women who are not used to heels, just remember to imitate the posture of wearing them, and most importantly, be conscious not to slouch!

Keep that Spine Straight: Back and Bulge

Despite being a fit and physically active person, I had never put much thought into my posture. I was of the opinion that working out alone would take care of all my health requirements. So, when I sat down, I got into a comfortably slouched position, stooping happily at my desk. This had not caused me any trouble for the longest time, so I continued to be blissfully careless. But for my second pregnancy, I had a rude awakening. After giving birth for the first time, the stomach muscles tend to loosen, and no amount of exercise can restore the original tautness. So, during my second pregnancy, I noticed that my bulge was bigger and heavier than the previous time. An unpleasant addition was the accompanying pain. My back hurt terribly, and eventually I had to do something that I had never done before—I had to take painkillers for it! And not just one, but a double dose just to be able to function normally.

When I visited my doctor, Dr Seema Jain, to complain about this, she told me while prescribing the medication: 'take care of your posture'. These five words struck me like a blow, and suddenly, I realised that my comfortable slouching position in my chair had led to this miserable state. By this time, I found sitting straight to be much more uncomfortable, since my body had become used to the slouching. But I knew what I had to do: my long-term health required that I become comfortable with this discomfort. This was easier said than done. The toughest part was the constant focus this required of me. I had to be aware of my posture at all times of the day. I did everything possible to keep myself in check, even changing my phone's wallpaper to a poster that read 'Sit tall, stand tall and walk tall'. Every time I looked at my screen, it reminded me to check my posture. After a few weeks of mindful and constant posture correction, sitting straight was no longer difficult, and good posture eventually became second nature to me.

Some specific exercise poses were invaluable in improving my posture and getting rid of my backaches. I practiced these religiously.

As with all these asanas, you can hold them up to 20 seconds, and up to 30 seconds when you get used to doing them. You can do each asanas two to three times. Breathing (inhaling/exhaling) will remain normal through the asanas.

Keep that Spine Straight: Back and Bulge

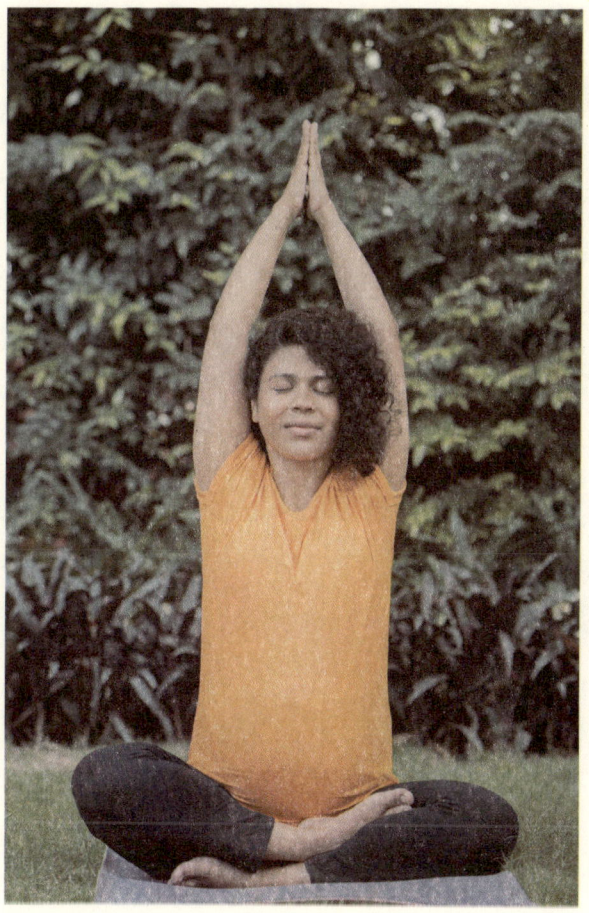

1: Sit comfortably with your knees in a crossed position. Hold your hands in a Namaste pose and lift them upwards. Stretch them towards the sky with your upper arms touching your ears. Pull your lower back upwards and feel the stretch in your entire back. Hold the position. Gently release.

Grow Your Baby, Not Your Weight

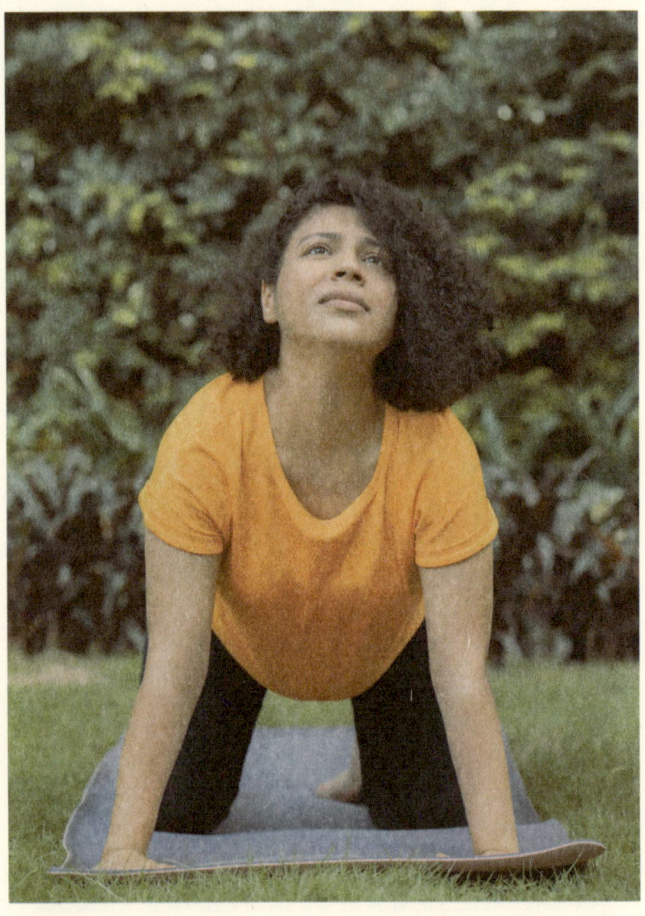

2: Cat Cow Pose: Kneel comfortably. Place your hands in front of you. Lower your back and, lifting your chest, look upwards. Hold this position. Gently release. Similarly, pull your back up and lower your chest, while looking downwards. Hold this position. Gently release.

Keep that Spine Straight: Back and Bulge

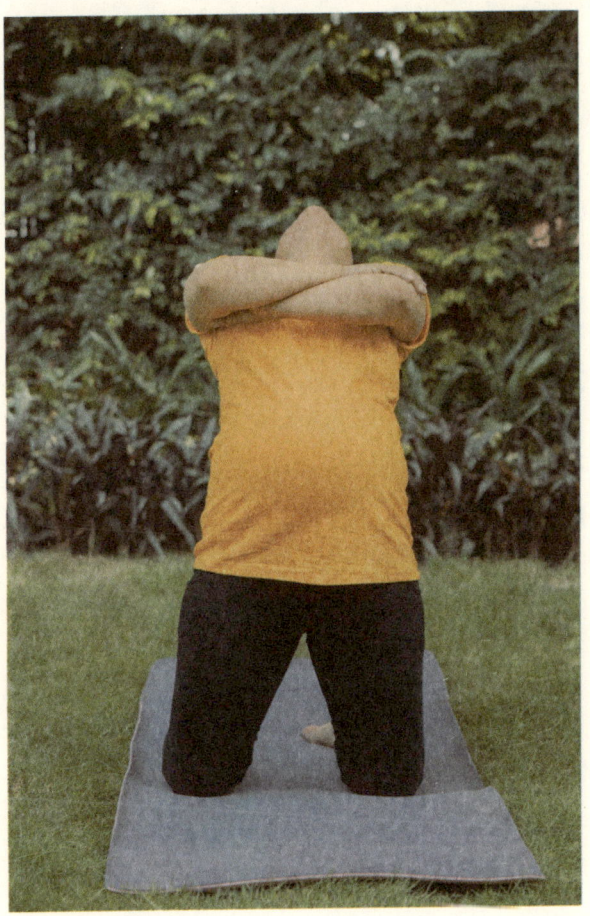

3: Again, kneel comfortably. Place your arms in front of your chest in a folded and overlapping position. Your elbows should be in alignment with your shoulders. Slightly lifting your chest, bend backwards. Feel the stretch in your entire back. Hold this position. Gently release.

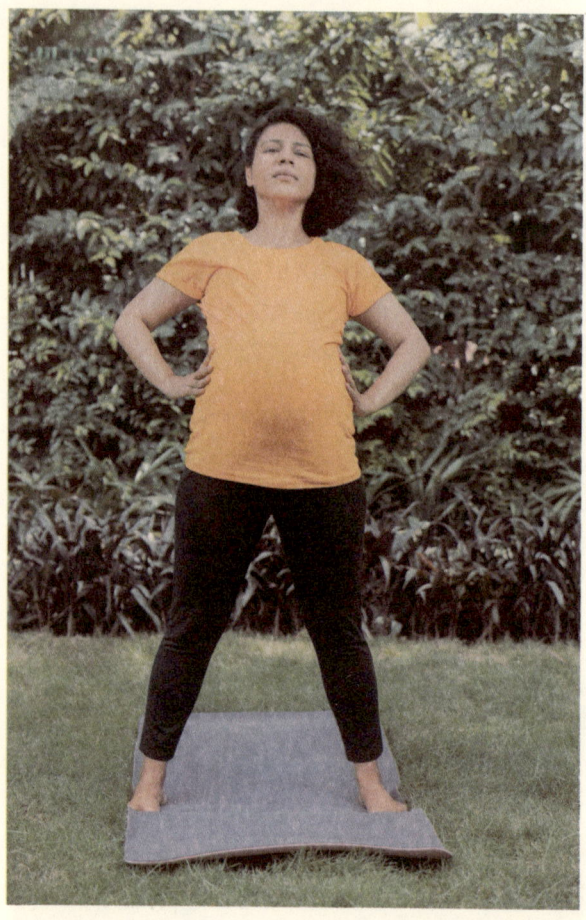

4: Stand with your legs open a bit wider than the gap between your shoulders. Place your hands on your sides. Now, carefully bend backwards with your shoulders stretched outwards. Feel the stretch in your entire back. Hold this position. Gently release.

Keep that Spine Straight: Back and Bulge

And of course, I can't emphasize enough how much I owe to the practice of squatting. It is an absolute game changer. From strengthening your lower body to correcting your posture, squats are the magic solution. Squats also have some of the most visible results after exercising, which definitely helps with motivation.

Whenever you find yourself slouching, remind yourself that your spine is the pillar that controls your body. Let it do its job of commandeering you with utmost efficiency. Hold your head high, throw your shoulders back, and walk as if the world is your red carpet. You will ooze confidence, and you will have earned all the praise you get for the work you have put into it.

7

SKYROCKET YOUR ENERGY LEVEL: SECOND TRIMESTER

And now, my dear reader, let us embark upon happier times together. To all of you who have come this far with me, thank you. We have been through some serious life changes together. From the initial shock and joy of realising that you are going to be a mother, to slowly but surely redesigning your life to suit your current needs, all with the utmost concern for the baby's health and safety—it has been a whirlwind. You have dealt with morning sickness, nausea, and a variety of aches. You have endured emotional upheavals, and sudden, irrepressible food cravings. You have accepted a changing body with grace

Skyrocket Your Energy Level: Second Trimester

and great anticipation. Now, it is time to welcome the second trimester with a gladdened heart. This trimester is the golden trimester of your pregnancy, so make sure that you enjoy it to the fullest.

After three months of constant checks and vigilance, your body and mind would have fallen into a well-set routine of healthy eating and conscious exercising. If you have put in the work so far, this will come easily to you now. Your body has been strengthened, as has your mind, making you more resilient than ever before. Now it is time to believe in yourself. You have worked hard and built faith in yourself; you can trust yourself to make the best decisions for you and your baby. Do not let doubt and uncertainty cloud your mind. Believe in your wisdom and instinct, and let your body guide your mind through a healthy and happy pregnancy.

The second trimester of pregnancy is sometimes called the 'honeymoon phase' of pregnancy, because these three months may be the easiest time of your journey. By this time, the problems of the first trimester, such as nausea and indigestion, have abated. Your body has become attuned to its new state. The hormonal imbalance is also brought somewhat under control, so you may start feeling like your old self, and your appetite makes a comeback. This is also a magical time of the 'quickening' of the womb. An old-fashioned expression, but it beautifully describes the time when your baby starts letting you know of its existence by moving inside you!

We have all heard about getting butterflies in our stomachs when we see our objects of desire. But one does not realise how literal that feeling can be when having a child. Quickening feels like strange wings fluttering inside the womb. To the less romantically inclined, this feeling can be compared to gassiness as well! In reality, it is the baby beginning to stir with life and vitality. By this time, the baby's webbed hands and feet have separated into little fingers and toes. She has a fully developed umbilical cord attached to the mother, and with time, she begins to exercise her newly formed muscles. As the trimester progresses, the movements become more pronounced, and towards the end of the fifth month, many mothers can feel the distinct kicks and jabs, and even hiccups, of their little ones inside the tummy.

Words fail to describe the pure and utter bliss of recognising movement in your womb. All at once, there is a realisation of an actual human being developing inside your body. This is when you begin to truly bond with your child, the child gifted to you by nature and nurtured with your own flesh and blood. The little kicks and bumps make your eyes brim with tears of pride and joy. This is your human, and you learn the meaning of true love from this little bundle to come.

Skyrocket Your Energy Level: Second Trimester

Many mothers-to-be continue to feel a sense of exhaustion and a general lack of energy. This can have physiological causes such as fluctuating blood pressure or thyroid imbalance. It is important to keep a check on all your vitals and consult the doctor for any possible disturbances. Sometimes, however, the cause for fatigue is rooted deeper in the mind. Society has conditioned us to believe that a pregnant woman is at a weakened and fragile state, and she needs constant rest. The stories we hear from our relatives, about sickness and exhaustion during their pregnancies, influence our own state of mind. It is crucial to recognise it for what it is: a mental conditioning that can easily be undone.

Instead of thinking about ways to combat fatigue, a cleverer solution is to focus on heightening our energy threshold. The body is a machine that follows the directions that the mind provides it with. It is the mind that needs to be trained in the most effective manner. You have the power to elevate your energy to a new level. All you have to do is make up your mind about it. Do not give in to negative self-talk and safeguard yourself from external negativity as well. Please remember that you are getting healthier every day. You are reaping the fruits of all the work you have put in. This is not the time to slow down. In fact, be more charged up than ever before. Believe that you have the ability to manifest your true potential and keep pushing your limits every day.

Routines are your best friends in life. Hopefully, your diet and exercise routines have already been set in place in the previous few months. But there are other, equally important aspects of life that need to be regularised as well, starting with sleep. Sleep hygiene is necessary for healthy living in general, but it becomes particularly urgent during pregnancy. Maintaining regular hours for waking up and going to bed is imperative. The quality of sleep is of greater importance than the number of hours. This is a good time to instil certain bedtime habits, such as not using the TV or digital screens in the bedroom and investing in good quality mattresses and pillows for sound sleep. Make your bed a sleep-only zone; your work should not be invited in there with you. Keep your working hours regulated, as far as possible, and don't let work bleed into every aspect of your life. Strive for balance in everything you approach.

It helps to plan out your day in advance, so that you get the opportunity to participate fully and be present at every moment of your day. We tend to spend far too much time on autopilot, not paying enough attention to our immediate circumstances and surroundings. Try to avoid that. 'Unseeing eyes' miss out on the little moments of joy that life brings us every day, and ultimately, it is these little moments of mindful presence that add up to a rich and fulfilling life. Plan to spend time with your family and loved ones every day. As a pregnant woman, you have a unique insight into the value of human existence and the pain and effort that goes into its creation. I made it a point to consciously enjoy my existence, with people around me that matter the most. Family bonding has a way of making you feel rejuvenated, and that is something I worked towards constantly.

Perhaps the most valuable practice that I started at this time was meditation and pranayama breathwork. The advantages of meditation are well-documented. Meditation helps control anxiety and emotional upheaval, improves quality of sleep, helps regulate blood pressure, and even helps to manage pain. Pranayam improves the respiratory system and helps build stillness and mindfulness. There is a large array of meditative practices, but I found a few specific ones most effective for me and worth talking about here.

1. Anulom Vilom: Sit comfortably with your legs crossed. Exhale completely and press your right nostril with your right thumb. Inhale from your left nostril and then press your left nostril with your fingers of the right hand. You can do each side 20 times, and later 50 times. Anulom Vilom helps in improving digestion and managing tension and anxiety.
2. Ujjayi Pranayama: Sit comfortably with your legs crossed. Constrict (tighten) your throat with your mouth closed. Start with an exhale and now inhale in one long and unbroken breath, creating a long

and sharp sound from your constricted throat. Hold this for 5 to 10 seconds and make sure to keep your head and neck straight. Then exhale normally. You can perform this pranayama up to 5 times. Ujjayi Pranayam helps in improving concentration levels and in calming the mind and body.
3. Bhramari Pranayama: Sit comfortably with your legs crossed. Cover your ears with your index fingers and your eyes with your fingers. As you inhale, create a humming bee like sound from your throat. Then exhale normally. You can perform this pranayama up to 10 times. Brahamari Pranayam helps control hypertension and improves the quality of sleep.

Meditating helped me bring order to my sleep cycle, including taking quick power naps. The post-afternoon slump is a well-known phenomenon that all office-going professionals are painfully aware of. Add to that the general weariness of pregnancy, and it is practically impossible to be at one's productive best in the afternoon. But a quick power nap can do wonders. Embrace these power naps in the afternoon with joy and enjoy the deep and peaceful slumber. This will recharge you and keep you fighting fit and ready to roar the rest of the day.

During pregnancy, one needs to be particularly careful and observant of one's emotional energy. Negativity in the mother can have unfortunate effects on the child in

Skyrocket Your Energy Level: Second Trimester

the womb. It is the mother's duty to try and remain as cheerful and positive-minded as she possibly can. Anger, hurt, worry, stress, tension, anxieties—these are a constant part of everybody's life. However, how much impact they are allowed to have on oneself depends on one's attitude. For my part, I told myself that I would treat stress the way I learnt about it in high school physics: as force exerted per unit area! I would not let it become a dark monster that preyed on my mind and impacted my well-being and that of my child. My meditation practice helped me enormously as it taught me to become an uninvolved observer of the many emotions that I faced every day, and to treat them as fleeting visitors only.

As a mother, you find out how important it is to forgive. Your child is new to the world; he or she is going to make mistakes as a part of growing up, and it will be your job to forgive lovingly and teach him or her right from wrong. I allowed myself to dip into my innate store of forgiveness from the time that I conceived. It helped me to overcome negativity and brush aside any hurt and frustrations that others caused me. I constantly reminded myself that I was in ultimate control of my own mind and my emotions. This gave me the power of resilience and freed me from the actions and judgements of others.

I chose to focus on my own passions and place unwavering faith in my convictions. An emotionally strong mother can guide her child well and protect him or her ferociously, when the need arises. I am often asked about my role models in life, and my response usually results in surprise. The truth is that I continue to be inspired everyday by the people around me, and their actions and choices. I choose joy and a positive outlook on life. My days are filled with resounding affirmations that I am strong and courageous. In fact, I have never needed to look outwards for inspiration or motivation. As women, we have an inexhaustible reservoir of strength within that we can tap into. We are the artists—making decisions to better ourselves and committing to this vision—as well as the art. True to these affirmations indeed, I have an unwavering focus. I am the artist and the art. I am the design!

I have always thought of myself as a conqueror, my own knight in shining armour. And as a mother, I knew that I would have to be the knight for another little soul looking up to me as well. This thought kept me going with renewed energy and passion. I sang a little childhood song to myself whenever I felt low—Savage Garden's 'Truly Madly Deeply'. I told myself, 'I love you more with every breath truly, madly, deeply,' and I meant every word of it. Loving myself taught me to love my children and my husband even more and gave me the zeal to be unstoppable.

Paulo Coehlo, in his celebrated book 'The Alchemist', said that when one truly aspires towards something, the

Skyrocket Your Energy Level: Second Trimester

entire universe comes together to give it to the person. And Shah Rukh Khan echoed this sentiment in his iconic dialogue in *Om Shanti Om, 'kehte hey ki agar kisi cheez ko dil se chaho, to poori kaynaat use tumse milane ki koshish mein lag jati hey.'* I am an ardent believer of this philosophy. I have seen it work many times in my own life. When I put in the effort and leave no stones unturned to achieve my goals, destiny works to assist me. And this mindset has helped me breeze through my pregnancies and transcend every minute of it.

So, I urge you to become the driver of your own destiny. You are powerful, and nature has made you flawless. You are entirely in charge of your life and all its facets. Perfection is whatever you define it to be. Believe in your ability to design your present and your future, and you can make the process of procreation as perfect as yourself. You will be the winner. And through you, so will your child.

Mindfulness and meditation helped me realise my potential, and during my pregnancy, no less. It was perhaps the most freeing experience of my life, one that I will always treasure. I continue to practice these lessons diligently, and you can, too. Honour yourself; hold yourself in high esteem. Happy evolution... happy skyrocketing of your energy levels!

8

REDISCOVER YOURSELF: FINAL TRIMESTER

Time flies—one day you are rejoicing over the news of your pregnancy, and the next day you are already six months into your journey. You have had some long days, many difficult days, and even some days of utter joy. But all of that is behind you already. You are in the last stretch of your pregnancy; the third trimester is here.

As the earth has ever-changing seasons, so do our lives. We have our joyful springs and summers, emotional monsoons, courageous autumns, and magical winters. But no matter what season one is in, impending motherhood brings with it a gust of spring. Scientific explanations cannot take away from the sheer miracle that is the evolution of

Rediscover Yourself: Final Trimester

life in the womb. The entire family becomes involved in readying the household to welcome its newest member, even as the sense of wonder washes over everyone.

The third trimester is a unique phase in your pregnancy journey. The other two trimesters have had their own ups and downs, but they have been somewhat predictable in their patterns. This final phase brings a little more uncertainty. By this point, you will have settled well into your pregnancy. Six months into it, your baby bump is now a proud proclamation to the entire world of your exciting journey. The routines that you have worked so hard to inculcate throughout your pregnancy are now well-established and you have gained mastery over your mind. Don't be surprised if you find an internal glow that dazzles you in the mirror. On a more functional level, though, you might find that mobility can sometimes be a challenge. You can no longer bend as you used to, and you start to forget what your feet look like because you haven't seen them in a while! However, this should not be an excuse for you to give up on your fitness routine. You can, and should, continue to be active. Just consult your doctor about any additional precautions that you might need to take at this time. Your legs will thank you for all the squats that you have been practicing, because at this point, the only way you can pick something up from the ground is by squatting down. I, for one, continued to go for slow jogs well into the last trimester because my overall health allowed me to. There are athletes who have been known to participate in the Olympics while pregnant, so there is no reason for you to stop your exercise routine either.

> **Dr Rekha on varicose veins:** Varicosities or varicose veins can occur in the legs and genital region for some pregnant women. These are caused due to the increased pressure applied by the uterus on the inferior vena cava: the large vein that carries blood from the legs back to the heart. Varicosities may cause itchiness and pain in the affected area. Pregnant women are advised to avoid standing for prolonged periods, but instead take frequent breaks to sit down. Keeping the legs in an elevated position may help with the discomfort. If the pain persists and becomes unbearable, women may use elastic stockings that squeeze the area and prevent varicosities.

For ages, there have been some rather restrictive norms for women who are expecting, many of them having no scientific backing whatsoever. For instance, women who are pregnant are advised to 'take it easy' because they are 'weak'. They are told not to drive a car at this time, even though this has no real impact on the pregnancy. In the Western world, it is not at all uncommon for women to drive themselves to the hospital when they go into labour, go through with the delivery, rest and recuperate for a few days, and then drive back home with the baby, all by themselves. This is a clear indication that there is in fact no problem with driving while you are expecting. So, do not let old-fashioned conventions tie you down, and continue to enjoy your long drives and commutes to work right up to your seventh month.

> **Dr Rekha on driving and travelling during pregnancy:** Women in India are often advised to avoid driving during pregnancy. However, this has no medical backing, and safe driving practices do not cause additional harm to the mother or baby. Extra caution may be observed while driving or travelling during the first trimester, which is a crucial phase of foetal development. It is best to maintain an even speed to avoid jerks and accidental impact while travelling. It is crucial to wear your seatbelt at all times, with the upper part of the belt sitting between the breasts and the lower part underneath the belly, in order to avoid undue pressure on the womb. According to the guidelines issued by the American College of Obstetricians and Gynaecologists, air travel is considered safe up to thirty-six weeks of gestation. International or long-haul flights may require frequent ambulation. Women should try to take short walks across the plane every hour of a long flight.
>
> It is advised that travel should be minimised in the third trimester, particularly after the seventh month, since labour can occur at any time, even before the due date.

Grow Your Baby, Not Your Weight

The challenges of the third trimester are rather curious. At this stage, you realise that your wardrobe has become mostly non-functional! There will be pretty dresses and gorgeous ethnic wear that simply don't fit you anymore. There are many who may become despondent about this. All at once, the reality of their increased size dawns upon them, making them morose. It does not help that others take it upon themselves to comment on pregnant women's bellies and overall weight at this time. These comments are sometimes well-meaning and solicitous, but can at times also be annoying and hurtful. This is when your own practice of self-love and resilience comes into play.

As a mother-to-be, you are responsible for creating and nurturing a new life inside you, a life that is almost ready to enter into this world. Think about it: when an apple is well ripened, it is red, rounded, and absolutely delicious. Is it not beautiful? What is an apple, really, but a carrier of the seeds of the tree, some of which fall to the ground to help bring about new life! The big and round apple keeps the seeds safe and is perfect for its function. Is an expecting mother's physical state really all that different? Her belly is growing her baby. It is, in quite literal terms, the baby's first home in this world. It keeps the baby safe and healthy, allowing the baby to grow until it is ready to come out into our world. The belly is a testament to the mother's infinite potential. Her body works as a vessel, a safe abode

Rediscover Yourself: Final Trimester

that provides succour to a new human being. It offers the best of health, nourishment, and vitality to the baby, and deserves respect and admiration for it. We are proud of our houses, and keep them well cared for, so, why should a mother feel anything but pride for her baby's home?

Society may value slimness over an out of shape belly, but in reality, you are in perfect shape for your present stage in your life. Even with my usual store of resilience and self-worth, I struggled with certain funny body image issues at the time of the final trimester. I kept feeling 'too big', and all the ill-fitting clothes in my closet seemed to haunt me. This became a greater issue in my second pregnancy, as my belly was significantly bigger this time around. I felt a bit anxious and complained about my shape to my husband Abhishek and my best friend Ravneet. They were both very supportive and tried their best to make me feel better. Abhishek reminded me of a crucial fact. He said, 'You have to remember that your belly is an indication of our child's health. The baby is getting bigger and stronger. Strong is good!' My best friend agreed and reminded me that it was the *baby* that was growing, not the belly. These words helped me to look at it from a different perspective, and I instantly felt much better. Indeed, I was big because so was my baby! I could feel a resurgence of my confidence, and with it returned my cheerfulness. I took my final trimester body out to shop for some pretty clothes that would make me feel as beautiful outside as my baby was within me. I no longer tried to 'hide' my belly—not that it was a realistic idea anyway. Instead, I chose clothes that allowed me to flaunt my impending motherhood to the world with grace and dignity. The older clothes in my closet could wait awhile.

Sometimes, the third trimester ends sooner than anticipated. The baby might be in a hurry to come out, and all the mother can do is to oblige. All the more reason to enjoy every moment of the final days of pregnancy. Years later, it will be these days that will remain deeply etched in your mind. You will not remember the nausea of the early days, or the aches and cramps of the second trimester. The third trimester, with its visual reminders of pregnancy, will be the most prominent. You will find yourself talking fondly about the many little incidents that took place at this time. The baby's kick that caused your belly to poke up at one place; the time your older child put her face to your belly to talk to her younger sibling; the long evenings you spent debating about baby names with the family; and the shopping sprees for the little one—these will remain cherished memories. Every special moment, both inside you and outside, will live on as stories that you will share with your little one. Make sure you participate fully in these moments, for these are treasured moments that do not return.

The final trimester also brings with it a host of new anxieties. As mothers, we start to worry about our little one's health and safety from the moment we become aware of the conception. In these final days, our anxiety peaks. All sorts of apprehensions about the baby's health post-birth haunt us. We worry with equal trepidation about the process of birthing itself. There is a creeping fear about whether everything will work according to plan, and whether we will be strong enough to handle the process. The mind has an uncanny ability to amplify hidden fears and catastrophise events. The causes of fear, anxiety, and frustration are as varied as mothers themselves. I personally began to dread the coming of night because sleeping had become increasingly difficult. I would toss and turn in bed, seeking a posture that would remain comfortable after the first fifteen minutes. If I lay straight, my back got stiff, and the constant pressure on my bladder made me get up three or four times a night for toilet runs. I often wished for this phase to pass quickly.

Eventually, what got me through was the conviction that everything was progressing perfectly. I reminded myself that my emotional state would have a direct impact on my baby's health and emotional state. I could not bear the thought of my child being a timid, fearful person, just because her mother had let herself dwell on irrational fears during pregnancy. That was by far my biggest worry, and so, ironically, I had to convince myself to stop worrying. What I learnt the hard way during my pregnancy was that, at the end of the day, you need to become your own counsellor.

Grow Your Baby, Not Your Weight

It is, of course, vital to have social support. I consider myself infinitely lucky to have my family. My parents, my husband, my best friend—they all made it their mission to keep me upbeat during my pregnancy. But the truth is that another person, even with the best of intentions, can only do so much. At the end of the day, you *have* to hold your own hand. Although this might sound sad, it is really an empowering realisation. You realise that ultimately, you have the greatest impact on and control over your own mind. You can direct your mind the way you choose, and so you can choose joy and peace. You do it for yourself and for your child.

Pregnancy is a time of creation and renewal. It is the best possible time to try your hands at a creative new practice. This can be anything—from painting to stitching, and house decor to origami. If you have a childhood hobby that was pushed to the backburner over the years, now is the time to revive it. Perhaps you enjoyed singing as a child, or you were a bookworm. Go out and get yourself art supplies or the new set of books you were eyeing for a while. Immerse yourself in creativity, and let your imagination run wild. There is a joy to creating new things with one's own hands that can rarely be surpassed. The strength and confidence you feel while engaging in a creative endeavour and the satisfaction with the end result is so rewarding.

Personally, I found my creative outlet in the writing

of this book. The idea of penning down my experiences and the lessons I learnt from both my pregnancies struck me towards the end of the third trimester of my second pregnancy. Earlier, during my stint with the sand mafia in UP, many people had told me that it would be a great idea to pen down my experiences. At that time, though, I did not feel the urge to do so. In fact, I was quite sceptical of the idea that I could write a book! Something changed during my pregnancy. All of a sudden, I was consumed with a new passion; I simply *had* to share my journey with the world. Mahatma Gandhi recorded his experiments with 'truth' in his book; with great humility, I wanted to make a record of my experiments with divinity. For that is exactly what childbirth is: a glimpse of the divinity accorded to ordinary human beings.

Doing something for yourself, now, will help you prepare for motherhood in the best possible way; it will remind you not to put yourself last when you look after your child's needs. As women, we are conditioned to be caregivers for everyone around us, and this increases manifold when our own children come into the picture. But even as we take care of everything the child needs, we are teaching them much more with our own actions than we realise. If a child sees that their mother is constantly sacrificing her own wants and desires, the child will grow up to take the mother for granted. That is not the sort of person you want to rear. It is crucial that children learn to share and to show respect from an early age, and respect begins with their behaviour towards their mother. A child who sees her mother take time off from parenting to pursue her own interests will grow up to become a more well-rounded person.

One of my favourite books is *The Secret* by Rhonda Byrne, in which the author says that the secret to a good life is to be grateful every step of the way. She talks about the laws of attraction in the context of gratitude, mentioning that the more you practice gratitude, the greater the reasons you will have to be grateful for. I have made the practice of gratitude the lodestar of my life and have experienced the truth of her words on many occasions. Gratitude is all about your attitude; you will always have much to be grateful for, should you choose to be so. Practicing gratitude by being thankful to the source of everything good and positive in my life has made me a kinder, more loving person. It has helped me become a reservoir of love; when my own cup is full, I can give with grace. Actions also have a way of coming back to you, and kindness usually begets kindness. Gratitude has made me happier and more peaceful, and this is something I intend to teach my children too.

As you near the end of your pregnancy journey, prepare yourself for the final part with courage and grace. Focus on the perfection that you embody and that you have absorbed through every step. Do not let fears and doubt

Rediscover Yourself: Final Trimester

cloud your mind, for they do not serve you. Your future will be as beautiful as the past and the present have been. Bask in the abundance that you hold within you—the little kernel of life that you have nurtured and grown into a full human being. You have lived your life to the fullest. In fact, you have lived two lives! You learned to believe in your own strength and wisdom. You now have the right to be exuberant about everything you have achieved. Your relentless, uncompromising zest for life has seeped into your baby, and its future will be shaped by it. Give yourself the pat on the back that you deserve and look towards the next stage with joy and excitement. The best times are about to begin!

9

JOURNEY'S FINALE: GIVING BIRTH

Well then, we are finally here. This is D-Day, the focal point of all the anticipation, preparation, and excitement for these nine months. The day has arrived when your baby is ready to see the light of day. It has been marvellous indeed, a life-altering journey. Hopefully, you have had the chance to grow in health and abundance, and rediscover yourself in countless ways. Your body, that fortress of strength and courage, is now ready for the final phase. This journey has been a marathon, and this is the ultimate hour.

Many women are overly concerned about their labour

Journey's Finale: Giving Birth

and delivery. For first-time mothers, there is much fear and apprehension regarding this final phase. One hears terrifying stories about the pain and gore that the process of birthing involves, some frightening enough to put some women off the idea of having children altogether! But if there is one thing I have learnt from being a mother twice over, it is that the scenarios we make up in our heads are far more appalling than reality. For one, the mind has a way of magnifying everything beyond normal proportions. It stretches an experience to monstrous degrees. And secondly, the mind invariably reaches the most unfortunate conclusions for any given circumstance.

All this could be further aggravated by an overload of information. We live in an age where Google allows us to find details about everything we could possibly want to know. While this has its own benefits, it can also lead to a lot of stress and suffering that may be avoidable. For both my pregnancies, I made a conscious decision to follow a need-to-know policy about everything that was happening to me. A lot of women put in enormous time and effort to familiarise themselves with every minute medical terminology associated with pregnancy and childbirth. They talk to friends and experts and make extensive contingency lists and plans to deal with different eventualities. The reality, though, is that there is not much that one can do to control circumstances beyond what I have already outlined in this book. Unnecessary medical knowledge will just give you more to worry about. I was determined to avoid that. My job already gives me a lot to be overly occupied with; I do not want my personal life to add to it. I followed this rule through labour and delivery as well, limiting the amount of information I consumed about the experience, and trusting my ability to cope with whatever may come my way. And I must say, this made the overall experience more enjoyable than frightening.

None of this is to say that you will not have to experience pain. Childbirth is a difficult process and leads to much physical suffering for the mother. It is often the most painful thing you will experience in your life. But the good news is that the pain lasts for a short time. On average, the duration of active labour lasts for around eight hours, from the time of increasing contractions to the complete dilation of the cervix. Even if your labour goes on for longer, remember, this is nothing compared to the nine months and the myriad pains and aches you have already experienced.

> **Dr Rekha on the labour and delivery:** Despite a growing trend among women to opt for a caesarean delivery, doctors (obstetricians) will usually advise normal delivery in most cases where the mother's pelvis is adequate for the baby. The weight of the baby becomes a deciding factor in whether normal delivery is possible, since a bigger

Journey's Finale: Giving Birth

> baby may require a C-section for the safety of mother and child. In case of complications in pregnancy, a C-section is advised. Natural birth is preferred by doctors as the post-delivery recovery is much quicker for the mother. In normal cases, mothers can attend to household chores within forty-eight hours of a natural birth. A caesarean is a surgery and requires a longer hospital stay of up to a week for recovery.
>
> In some cases, a mother may be having a breech baby in late pregnancy. This is a situation where the head of the baby is upwards and the legs are downwards. This is a malposition of the baby during pregnancy, which may need a C-section. A transverse position of the baby may also require C-section delivery. Experienced obstetricians may be able to assist the mother to deliver a breech baby naturally, however, in most cases, a caesarean may be recommended to avoid risks.

For my first child, I was determined to have a normal delivery. But things don't always go exactly according to plan. My due date came and passed, but I felt no contractions at all. I had had a full term of gestation, yet my baby was not showing much interest in coming out! The next day we spoke to my doctor, who advised going in for induced labour, as late term pregnancies can have increased risks for the mother and child. Soon, I found myself in the hospital bed, an IV injecting labour-inducing drugs into my body. These are medications that initiate contractions in the uterus to prepare it for labour, when the body does not do so by itself. One unfortunate effect of induced labour is that unlike in natural labour, where contractions increase gradually, the effect is abrupt. All of a sudden, my uterus was awake and at work, spasming and contracting, determined to push the baby out. The pain hit me all at once and continued through the twelve hours of my labour. But then again, what does not kill you makes you stronger. My inner Gabbar Singh reminded me, '*jo darr gaya, samjho marr gaya*', and I could not contradict that!

Those twelve hours were tough. The pain made me howl. What kept me going was my inner grit and resilience. I have always believed myself to be a fighter, and I was not going to let myself down at that crucial moment. This was a test of patience, and time seemed to crawl by. But I kept telling myself that victory was at hand, and that this moment, too, would pass. Another important pillar of strength that got me through this was my husband Abhishek. Abhishek is a true son of the soil, a dyed-in-the-wool desi. His true traditional roots come to the forefront in moments of crisis. As my howling continued, he came into the room, rubbed my back, then held my hand and started chanting the *Hanuman Chalisa*! Even through the pain, my initial reaction to this was irritation. My rational mind wanted to shout at him and retort that religious chants could not improve

Journey's Finale: Giving Birth

the situation. But this was soon overtaken by other feelings. I realized that my husband had invoked something much deeper than mere words of comfort; he was channeling his traditional faith in divinity to help me conquer this trying hour. Modernity had given way to generational wisdom. He had somehow understood that what I needed was not mere physical reassurance, but emotional succour, and this was his way of providing it to me.

And then, it was time for the home run. I was taken into the delivery room, and the doctors worked on me. Let me tell you something that we rarely acknowledge: giving birth is a joint exercise. The mother has to undergo the physical exertion, but she has an entire team of doctors, nurses, and technicians around her at all times, guiding her and cheering her on at every step of the way. The patience, zeal, and stamina that the birthing team exercises is beyond incredible. By the end of it, the doctor and the nurses are almost as exhausted as the mother herself! The final moments of giving birth are a blur. Being placed in a slanting bed, I did not have a clear view of the birthing. But at one point, I watched in amazement and horror as a gush of blood was expelled out of me all over my doctor's face. I shall never forget her absolute lack of reaction. She did not falter for even a second, her focus undiminished, with no change of expression on her face. Birthing is a messy process, during which the mother is vulnerable and highly sensitive. Even a slight show of disorientation on the doctor's part can affect her negatively. I will forever be in awe of the professionalism and care my doctor, Dr Seema Jain, exhibited that day. Truly, she is a hero.

Your gynaecologist/obstetrician has shared your pregnancy journey from the initial stages, assisting you, soothing you, and keeping you safe and healthy. She has come to know your body and your baby almost as well as you do, perhaps even better. This is no longer a mere professional acquaintance; it is a relationship that has been cultivated and nurtured with time and patience. Medicine is a noble profession, and gynaecology is, perhaps, the crown jewel. These doctors assist with the miracle of birth. My baby was in my arms because of my doctor's ceaseless support. I can never thank her enough for it.

And all at once, it is done. You have given birth. Your baby has arrived. It is a surreal moment. After my first time, my doctor announced, 'It is junior Durga!' and the nurses brought her to me. I was in a haze, and for some time, nothing seemed to make sense. I did not have an immediate reaction on seeing my child; it was almost as if I had gone numb. The nurse told me, 'You can kiss her,' and my mind spent a few milliseconds wondering where I should kiss her, on her forehead, her cheek, or her lips! And then it dawned on me. This was my child, my baby who I had held in my belly for nine months, creating her

Journey's Finale: Giving Birth

with my own flesh and blood. She had been with me all this while, but now that she was before my eyes, it felt different, more real than it had ever been. I had felt her presence inside me before, but now, as I looked at her, I fell in love, hard and fast. Moments ago, my body had been a volcano, erupting with pain, but now that pain had been pushed millions of miles underneath, and all that remained was absolute bliss.

Abhishek had been waiting for us outside the room, presumably with some impatience. The nurse took the baby to him. I later heard that his first reaction on seeing our child had been to take her into his arms and inspect the shape of her head and the number of fingers and toes she had, just to make sure that everything was in perfect condition. How the nurse must have laughed at this, and the amusement was well deserved too, after the battle she had just been through! I will never cease to wonder at the many, tiny but stark differences in how men and women react. Abhishek, through all his joys and anxieties, had had the most utilitarian reaction possible, examining the child's physical aspects. No wonder the French say, 'vive la différence'!

After an hour or so, I needed to use the washroom. I told my doctor so, and she simply told me, 'Okay, get up and go!' This left me stunned for a moment. I had just given birth, and my doctor thought me capable of using the loo by myself! This was some confidence on her part, considering the storm that I had just been through. But it gave me the boost I needed, and I went ahead. It was wonderful to start moving towards normalcy so soon. Once I was back, and my mother was in the room, she asked my doctor the most mother-like question possible—what I could eat. The doctor reassured her that since it had been a normal delivery, I could eat all normal food with ease. My mother turned to me gleefully and said, 'See I told you, normal leads to normal,' making the doctor smile. Mothers, I tell you. They have a way of bringing a universe of comfort with them in the most natural manner possible.

It did not take long for the attention to be deflected from me. Soon, the room swarmed with family and friends, and even strangers. We Indians love childbirth, and flock to see the new baby with little concern about relations to the family! Everyone first rushed to the baby, and then, only reluctantly, came to me afterwards. Clearly, the woman of the hour had made her position as Chief Guest well known. But I could not complain. As people stood around her, showering her with compliments, I basked in their reflected glory. The baby was the star, but some telepathic connection allowed me to feel every bit of happiness and praise directed at her. This was the most beautiful moment: she was perfect, and she was mine.

There you go, you have done it. Bravo, and bravo! You have reached the finish line with finesse. You have created

Journey's Finale: Giving Birth

an impeccable work of art. You have given birth to a child, and in the process, *you* have been reborn, reincarnated in the sacred role of mother. Enjoy every moment of it, you have earned it.

> **Dr Rekha on postpartum care:** Regular antenatal visits with the gynaecologist are crucial and must not be avoided. These checkups allow the doctor to track the new mother's health and detect any problems at the outset. The first checkup is scheduled six weeks post-delivery, and it includes screening for infections and normal shrinkage of the uterus to pre-pregnancy levels.
>
> Post-delivery, it is advised to use contraception in order to ensure adequate spacing between subsequent pregnancies.
>
> Some mothers may require episiotomy during natural birth. This is a small incision made in the perineum to assist in the birth of the child. In such a case, it is important to maintain hygiene in the area after delivery, and to keep the area clean and dry. Application of betadine ointment after using the toilet is recommended.
>
> Hygiene needs to be maintained in breastfeeding as well, with cleaning done after each feed. This will prevent milk crystallisation in the nipple area that can lead to dryness and painful cracks.
>
> Some women face postpartum blues which may last a

few hours to a few days after delivery. This is characterised by sudden mood swings. This can be handled with proper family support and care. In rare cases, this might turn severe and become postpartum depression. This is a psychiatric complication that may be exacerbated by external impetus such as family troubles. It will require intervention by a trained psychiatrist, who may prescribe medication, including antidepressants, for the mother for several months.

10

SAME DESTINATION: DIFFERENT JOURNEYS

Have you ever experienced that vaguely unsettling feeling of walking down a familiar road, yet noticing that things are not exactly as you remember them to be? You know that you are in well-trodden territory, but things are not quite the same as before. This is a surprisingly universal human experience that often gets overlooked. Think about the time when you went back to your hometown after a long time, and though you could recognise every pathway, every nook and pebble in your neighbourhood, something kept niggling at the back of your mind, pointing out the multiple little ways that your all-too-familiar surroundings had changed. Or maybe it was the time when you met a childhood friend after a hiatus of a decade, and though your dear companion of the past brought back familiar sensations and warm fuzzy feelings, you could somehow sense that he or she was not quite the same person that you had known all those years ago. Having more than one pregnancy is a similar scenario. You know what to expect, you know the broad layout of the road ahead of you, but it will most certainly not be exactly the same journey that you have previously had.

How my second child came into being is a story of unexpected turnabouts in itself. I had had Dania five years previously and had enjoyed and struggled in equal parts through the motherhood experience. Abhishek and I were still at a nascent stage in our respective careers when we became parents, and the next few years had been spent in strengthening our professional foundations while juggling parenthood. While we had both wanted a sibling for Dania, the timing had never been quite right. Now, in Dania's fifth year, we were no longer seriously considering a second child.

This is the point I was at mentally, when I had one of my regular checkups with my gynaecologist, Dr Seema Jain. While conversing casually, she asked me whether we were considering having another child, as she thought that delaying it much longer might not be a very safe idea. I told her that my little one was five already, and that we thought a six-year gap between siblings might be a little too much. My husband and I were also getting busier, and we felt that we might not be able to do justice to a second child at this point.

Dr Jain heard me out and then laughed. 'Six years is *not* too large an age-gap between siblings by any count. I have two children myself, and they have a difference of six years too. I never saw *that* creating a problem!' She told me that both she and her husband were doctors, with entirely unpredictable schedules and gruelling working hours, but they had worked together to ensure that both their children had a healthy, well-rounded childhood. 'It is the will that really matters,' she reminded me, 'and the logistics tend to take care of themselves.' Her reassuring words set me thinking more intently about this problem. It is true that having siblings is a wonderful blessing. Siblings have each other's backs when the going gets rough, and can learn vital skills like patience, sharing and empathy from dealing with each other. As parents too, we can sleep a little easier knowing that our children need never be entirely alone. The more I thought about it, the more it seemed like a good idea.

I went back home that day and brought up the issue with Abhishek. He was willing to stand by whatever decision I made, considering, as he very sagely pointed out, that it was *I* who would have to do the lion's share of the work. I was already rather certain about the direction in which my wishes lay. Dr Jain, bless her, had given me the nudge that I required, and I was now ready to take the plunge. So, the decision was made, and only a few weeks later, the journey began.

This time I was infinitely better prepared. I knew what to expect, the roadblocks to anticipate and the precautionary measures to take from the get-go. As a result, my level of anxiety was significantly lower this time around. During my first pregnancy, I had suffered from occasional bouts of breathlessness. Looking back, I realised that most of it had stemmed from my worries and insecurities; my anxiety had manifested through shortness of breath. For my second pregnancy, I put a lot more effort into my mental and emotional balance. I developed a habit of meditation and chanting that helped assuage my worries and fears. The ancient practice of chanting is sometimes laughed at as religious superstition, but modern science has proven, beyond doubt, the physiological benefits of meditation. It helps calm your central nervous system and regulate your blood pressure, helping bring about a state of emotional quiescence. Meditation allowed me to feel centred and remain unfrazzled through these days.

For my second pregnancy, I embraced the 'planning and systems' geek inside me. I decided that I would plan out each of my days to the minutest detail, one day prior. Soon enough, I realised that I was never going to have enough

Same Destination: Different Journeys

time to get as many things done as I wanted to. I sometimes sent up quick little huffs of frustration, complaining to the Lord that He had made a mere twenty-four-hour day, rather than the more reasonable forty-eight! I knew that I had to give supreme importance to my health, and so I began waking up a little earlier than before so that I could make time for my morning walk and yoga practice before diving headlong into the myriad responsibilities of the typical workday. I refused to allow myself cheat days from meditation, squeezing in a minimum of five minutes after waking up or before going to bed, no matter how tired or unwilling I felt in the moment. It took a few months, but eventually, this became second nature to me. Now, I cannot imagine going through a day without finding a little gap in which to meditate. This was another of the many good habits that I imbibed on my journey to motherhood.

Abhishek and I had both been clear about one thing from the very beginning—we were not going to fail our first child in our bid to prepare for and bring up the second one. Dania was going to continue getting all the love, affection, time, and support that she deserved from her parents, no matter how many siblings came along, or how hectic work became. During my second pregnancy, I saw to it that Dania did not feel left out or excluded; she was going to be as much an active part of this journey as her parents.

My daughter made me proud. After finding out that her mummy was bringing her a little sister (or brother!), she assumed the role of my little helper with alacrity. Whenever I needed some assistance with daily household chores or anything else, my sweet little assistant was only too willing to oblige. I watched with wonder and pride as my little girl became kinder, more patient, and more cooperative than she had ever been. She would massage my aching legs with lotion, draw the curtains if the sun felt too bright for my eyes, and bring me a glass of water whenever I asked for it. She did as much as her little hands allowed, sometimes more. I once found her trying to fold the sheets and make the bed in the morning, so that mummy could rest her back for a while. I knew that my baby-to-come was going to be in good hands with her older sister.

Not that Dania did everything merely out of love for her parents. She is a master negotiator, my little one. Even as she went about helping around the house, she never forgot to mention that she expected some goodies or a few extra minutes on the iPad as rewards for her good behaviour. For the most part, though, she just wanted her parents' love and attention a little more than usual. That was all it took to encourage my daughter to become a more responsible, more obedient child, and I certainly could not ask for more.

There were a few things that went slightly awry with the second pregnancy. The scariest experience was the

Same Destination: Different Journeys

bleeding in the first trimester, induced through physical overexertion. I learnt my lesson, though, and remained much more careful throughout the rest of the months. Though my weight gain was the same compared to the first time, my belly acquired a more distended shape. Overall, however, I remained within the permitted levels of safe weight gain, so I was not too worried.

I suffered from a higher degree of acidity and heartburn in my second pregnancy. During the first trimester, I would spend several days at a stretch feeling uncomfortably bloated with frequent acid reflux. My doctor recommended digestive medication, but the effects were temporary. One day, after a particularly irritating bout of heartburn, I took out some cucumbers from the refrigerator and started chomping on them. The cooling sensation of the vegetable soothed my food canal, and I enjoyed the feeling so much that I started eating three or four cucumbers every day. I quickly realised that these veggies were actually helping to keep my acidity at bay much better than my medication had. So, it came about that I became a daily ingester of up to a half kilo of cucumbers, sprinkled with pink salt and a spritz of lemon. My family members watched me enjoy this simple delicacy and quickly followed suit. Now, our household tends to go through around one and half kilos of cucumber a day. The clear skin and sturdy digestion are welcome side effects.

Another tasty and healthy snack that I gorged on to

help with acid reflux was dahi tadka. It is a surprisingly easy dish to whip up within minutes, and it pairs wonderfully with rotis. The meal is sumptuous and filling and brings immense relief. All you have to do is to throw some desi tadka in a bowl of curd.

Another unfortunate side effect that caused me much annoyance in my second pregnancy was sudden cramps in my calf muscles in the middle of the night. A muscle pull in the calf is a fairly common problem in pregnancy, particularly during the second and third trimesters. The calf muscles contract suddenly, sending a piercing pain through the legs. It is particularly uncomfortable because of its unexpected commencement when a person is sound asleep. I would often wake up with the sensation of being stabbed in my leg and feel like I was handicapped and unable to get onto my own feet. Ironically, one of the most effective measures to alleviate cramps in calf muscles involve standing straight with added weight on the affected leg. This became far too difficult to try with my baby bump, so I practiced rotational exercises for the calf muscle while being in the same lying down position. This process quickly relieved the muscle pull without the need to stand up. The result was the instant disappearance of the sharp pain, and I was able to drift back to sleep.

My family continued to play the most crucial role of keeping me active and upbeat. For both my pregnancies I

Same Destination: Different Journeys

had decided to try and maintain my usual lifestyle as far as possible. During my second pregnancy, this was slightly more difficult, because I now had added responsibilities at work, along with another child to look after at home. To top that, we were in the process of renovating our house in order to make exclusive space for Dania. I insisted on being involved in the planning and supervising process. Sometimes, things would inevitably fall through the cracks, but I had people around me who stepped up and helped me sail through. My sister-in-law, Archana, is a dear friend to me, closer to a sister by blood than by marriage. She swooped in and relieved me of all my social obligations in the later part of my pregnancy. Whenever there was any festivity to be organised, or any family get-together to be planned, she took it upon herself to ensure that everything went smoothly with minimal involvement on my part. And she refused to take extra credit either! 'Oho bhabhi, you just leave it to me and focus on the babies,' she would say, and the next thing I knew, another successful social event would have been organised without a hiccup!

Life tends to throw you curveballs when you least expect them. For me, this came in the way of an unforeseen and unusual situation in the second pregnancy. I found out from my regular ultrasound, at around the thirty-second week, that my baby was in breech position. This meant that the baby had its head in the direction away from the birthing canal. This was a cause for concern, because babies in breech position usually turn around by this time in the pregnancy, facilitating a natural birth. But my doctor assured me that there was still time for the baby to turn. The next few weeks I kept praying fervently for my baby to spin around, but during the next scan a month later, she was still breech. This was most distressing, because I was set on having a natural birth this time around as well, and the breech position would make this nearly impossible.

As usual, my family jumped in to become my shield. My mother, with her own brand of dismissive no-nonsense attitude, told me not to overthink the situation. 'We'll see how things work out, now stop worrying.' My father started including a prayer for my baby turning around in his daily worship. '*Bachcha, seedha ho ja*,' he would say, and I would invariably wonder who it was that he was sending his pleas to, the Almighty or the little baby! We were ready to try all sorts of tricks and hacks at this point, so long as they did not pose any danger to us. Somebody had suggested playing music to the baby near the lower belly, so that the baby may turn around to be able to hear better. Dania, armed with her newly practiced song 'Five Hundred Miles', appointed herself the household musician. She would put her face next to my belly and hum the song incessantly, driving me to distraction, as much with love as with annoyance! My father's acquaintance suggested that I talk to the baby, but

Same Destination: Different Journeys

I delegated this responsibility to Abhishek. He would get on his knees and knock on my belly, as if it were the door to a house, and tell the baby '*Aaja oye, neeche aaja!*' And so proceeded our joint endeavour to get the baby to 'palat'!

I did not have high hopes, though; I had not felt any movement in my belly that would suggest that the much-anticipated turning had taken place. So, imagine my astonishment and absolute delight when, having gone in for my last scheduled scan, I was informed that the baby was no longer in breech position! I have had many occasions for sudden joy and victory in my life, but I can say without an ounce of uncertainty that this was the biggest, most important piece of good news that I had ever experienced, or ever will. My family soon joined in the celebration, each member claiming that his or her technique had worked its magic. I will always wonder what happened. Was it some obscure, scientific process, or the sheer human willpower of the joined psyches of my family that had led to this frankly miraculous turn? I suppose we will never know for sure. But if ever I had harboured doubts about the power of the human mind, those have disappeared for good.

By and by, it was time to bring our newest family member into the world, and into our household. As the due date approached, my mother started packing my hospital bag for me. This took me back to the first time, and once again, I wondered at the miracle that is childbirth. Here we were, packing with so much love and care for a person who had not even come into being outside of me. This time around, my sense of wonder was doubled when I saw Dania helping her grandmother pack with so much enthusiasm. History was repeating itself, yet the experience was different, for the previously much awaited little being was now doing her bit to welcome the newcomer.

And then The Day arrived. It was a strange case of déjà vu for me, as if I were reliving the day six years ago when Dania had come into this world. There was the induction of labour, the wait, the increasing pain, and the edge of delirium. As if to remind me that this was, in fact, a new day with a new person, my contractions decided to amp up a notch, sending daggers of pain to my back. But I was familiar with the routine, and I knew for a fact that a real treasure, more precious than all the gold in the world, awaited me at the other side of the pain. Eventually, the long night came to a close, the anxious wait was over, and my little bundle of joy, my little Digara, was in my arms. All was right with the world.

11

PREGNANCY AND CHILD REARING: IT'S A FAMILY AFFAIR

In today's professional world, teamwork is highly regarded. The more efficient a team player you are, the higher is your value to the organisation. If there is one thing parents understand, it is that it indeed takes a village to raise a child. The role of the family becomes crucial from the conception itself. The initial reaction of the family to the news can have a lasting impact on the expecting mother. I count myself most fortunate on the family front. My family members are my rocks, my pillars that get me through all sorts of rough patches and turbulent times, and my pregnancies were no different.

Grow Your Baby, Not Your Weight

Pregnancy brings women together in a shared empathy, since women naturally tend to have a more instinctive understanding for a fellow mother-to-be. A woman who is expecting looks to her female friends for companionship, and older ladies in her family for support and advice. But this does not mitigate the role of the men in our lives during this phase at all. A family attains fulfillment through the combined efforts of men and women, fathers, brothers and husbands as much as mothers and aunts. The lack of empathetic male support cannot be an enviable situation for any mother-to-be.

When it comes to pregnancy, the biggest source of support and comfort that a woman can hope for is, of course, her husband. He is her partner in this journey, every step of the way. The woman draws strength and confidence from her partner, and pregnancy is a time when she needs a lot of both. As Indians, we tend to frown upon any form of overt display of affection between spouses. The marital relationship of love and companionship is expected to be discreet and kept behind closed doors. But pregnancy is a special time, and a relaxing of reserve between spouses is quite common. In my case, for example, both Abhishek and I prefer to remain rather formal in public settings. This saw a significant change during my pregnancies. Abhishek, always a caring husband, took his new role as caregiver very seriously indeed. He insisted on holding me by the hand

Pregnancy and Child Rearing: It's a Family Affair

whenever I got out of a car or a plane, or even walked on a slightly uneven pathway. Any sort of elevation at all, and he would be there, lending me his arm, long before my bump had become visible! His overprotective attitude made me laugh, and I would tease him that he was announcing my pregnancy to the world much too early through his behaviour. But in reality, this tiny gesture of his conveyed to me a world of emotional care and support, helping me tackle the hurdles of everyday life. I knew that it was a hand that would hold me and comfort me throughout my life, and this knowledge left me feeling safe and content, ready to conquer my pregnancy together with him. After all, I was having the baby, but *we* were entering parenthood together.

My father, too, had an active role to play in keeping me afloat during my pregnancy. From the very beginning, Papa has been my greatest friend, philosopher, and guide in my professional and personal life. It is his experience and wisdom that I look to whenever I feel stuck in a difficult work situation. During both my pregnancies, I remained determined not to compromise on any of my work commitments, including my personal passion projects. For some time now, I have been actively involved in mentoring aspiring UPSC candidates and appearing as a motivational speaker at different student communities, including as a part of the TED platform. These engagements take up an immense amount of time and energy. Before each occasion, I spend at least two to three days on intense brainstorming sessions to curate the best possible advice and experience that I can then share with my audience. Through my pregnancies, as at other times, my father remained my personal coach and advisor, helping me draft the best possible speech every single time. It was almost as if he was the life coach to the motivational speaker! Pregnancy often leads to added exhaustion, and at times, it was his relentless energy and persuasion, more than my own zeal, that kept me going.

Unlike many other fathers, mine has always been particular about the homemaking part of life. During my pregnancies, it was my father who became meticulous, bordering on obsessive, about ensuring that I was served fresh food only, no exceptions. Any reheated leftovers would go to other family members, including himself, but my baby and I were only getting freshly cooked food every day. He sometimes drove the family up the wall with his insistence, but I could not have been more thankful.

When it comes to womanly care, I was lucky to have three older ladies looking after me, my grandmother, my mother and my mother-in-law. After the birth of my older daughter Dania, there are now four generations of women living in our household: Dania, myself, my mother, and her mother, our eighty-five-year-old badi nani. During my pregnancies, I never wanted for motherly care; in fact, I

Pregnancy and Child Rearing: It's a Family Affair

had my pick of mothers waiting to guide and support me as I needed!

My mother is the Iron Lady of the house. She is the most no-nonsense person ever and believes in giving it to you as it is, no sugar coating necessary. She is also a great believer in tough love. Her disposition is that of a drill sergeant, and she used this to the fullest to make sure that I was keeping fit during pregnancy. She made it her foremost duty to wake up at quarter to six every morning and wake me up as well, so that we could then go for a forty-minute morning walk. I do not recall even a single day when she let me skip the walk; I clearly did not have much choice but to stay fit and trim throughout! Ma made certain that I did not use my pregnancy as a reason to get out of engagements. With her around, tiredness was not a viable reason for skipping anything. She was my source of strength—she scolded me into believing that pregnancy was not a handicap, and definitely not a reason to allow myself to slack professionally or otherwise. If I ever tried to bow out of a social event or meeting using my pregnancy as an excuse, she was the first to push me out the door, telling me, '*kuch nahi hua hai tujhe.*'

Ma's tough love spilled over into my dietary habits as well. I remember an incident from my first pregnancy, when I spent a few days in my parents' house. I slept with ma one night and woke up around two in the morning due to a sudden, intense craving for food. It was one of those strange pregnancy cravings that you just *have* to satisfy, no matter what. I decided to try my luck with my mother, because I wanted some kind of delicacy at that hour. I woke her up, planning to use my pregnancy card to coax her into getting to the kitchen and whipping something up. No such luck. Without so much as moving a muscle, my mother informed me that she had kept a big, fat banana on the bedside table for me, and I should have that and quietly go back to bed! Imagine my distress: my mother had actually anticipated this eventuality and prepared a healthy snack in advance, so that poor pregnant me would be left with one measly banana!

We have a very distorted, dated idea about the relationship that a wife shares with her mother-in-law. Hindi soap operas have ignited the popular imagination with stories of scheming mothers-in-law torturing their poor, innocent bahus. The reality is often far removed from this gory picture. In my house, for example, my mother-in-law holds a place of reverence and love. I value her goodwill and put a lot of store in her advice. Our bonds of love came to be tested in my second pregnancy, when I made a miscalculation of not listening to my body in how much I was working out. One day, while still in the first trimester, I went for a jog in the morning, attended my dance class in the evening, and then followed it up with a slow casual evening stroll with my mother. I did not realise it in the process, but I had clearly overdone the physical exertion. This resulted in sudden, profuse bleeding, giving me quite a scare. I got in touch with my doctor, who scheduled an emergency ultrasound. Thankfully, the scans revealed that no serious damage had been done to the baby, though the doctor advised me strongly against any exertion for the next seven to ten days.

> **Dr Rekha on miscarriage risk and prevention:** It is important to understand that miscarriages can occur in healthy women and should not be stressed about unduly. A woman who has had a previous miscarriage does have a higher chance of suffering from it again. But by following the doctor's advice, it is entirely possible for a woman to carry to term and give birth to a healthy baby despite previous miscarriages. Almost fifty percent of all miscarriages occur due to chromosomal defects. Certain health conditions in the mother may also increase her risks of having a miscarriage. Some of these issues include diabetes, hypothyroid, progesterone deficiency, autoimmune diseases, uterine defects, etc. Drug abuse may also significantly raise the risk of miscarriage. Most miscarriages occur in the first trimester of pregnancy, and the probability of a miscarriage reduces somewhat after the first trimester.

Grow Your Baby, Not Your Weight

Back home, I felt a lot of trepidation and embarrassment while narrating the incident to my mother-in-law. I felt guilty and prepared myself for some well-deserved rebuke and disappointment from her. But her next words took me entirely by surprise. She said, 'You know, this is actually a good thing. In our village, we consider this to be a sign of the strength of the baby, when despite the bleeding, the baby remains in perfect condition.' What warmth, what profound comfort I felt in her words that day. Her simple, rustic beliefs had done more to soothe my anguish than any expertise could ever have done. I learnt two great lessons that day: overdoing anything is not a good idea, and I am blessed to have the most loving, kind mother-in-law anyone could ever hope for.

When Dania arrived, she was ensconced in the love and care of not one, but four mothers. This is a privilege that few children ever enjoy. There was never any dearth of maternal care for her, and I never had anything to worry about. This was perhaps the single biggest reason that allowed me to get back to active duty after just thirty days of my delivery, even though the usual duration of maternity leave is six months post-delivery. I would express the breast milk before going and made sure it was sufficient. Sometimes, the multiplicity of mothers led to hilarious incidents. For example, the baby needs to be administered a plethora of vaccines in the first few months of her birth. In most

Pregnancy and Child Rearing: It's a Family Affair

families, the norm is for the parents to bring the child to the hospital for the vaccination. In Dania's case, she was lucky that when both her parents left for work, her grandmother was available to do the routine medical rounds. On one of these rounds, ma went to the hospital dressed in a bright purple kurti that was most fetching on her, Dania a tiny bundle in her arms. She must have cut quite an interesting picture in a sea of younger mothers. Soon, one of these ladies came up to her and asked her hesitantly whether the baby in her arms was her child. My mother had a good laugh, before replying '*Iske maa baap mere bacche hain!*' (Her parents are my children!) We were all very tickled to hear her story afterwards, and when I teased her that it was really just her kurti that had made her look so young, she retorted immediately with 'I always look young anyway!'

As Dania grew a little older, the alliances in the household became increasingly clear. My little daughter had found her closest friend and confidant in our badi nani. The age difference wasn't much at all—a mere eighty years! Ours is a family of tough personalities and firm minds, and with the great divergence of opinions we all harbour, our house is a constant battlefield. We give the Mahabharata a run for its money with our disagreements, and it is a matter of perpetual awe to me that we don't send a member or two to the hospital for injuries after each of these! But if there were ever two people who had one heart and one

Grow Your Baby, Not Your Weight

soul, they are Dania and badi nani. In all the six years of her existence, I have never once seen my daughter disagree with her badi nani on any matter whatsoever. They are each other's partners in crime, providers of mutual alibis, and staunch defenders of each other. It is adorable to see the two of them functioning as a unit.

It is the unwavering support from my family that helped me battle many of the strange myths regarding pregnancy. One popular myth claims that an expecting mother who goes outside the house during a lunar eclipse will end up birthing a child with a cleft lip. More stringent versions of the belief declare that the mother should desist from eating or drinking anything at all for the duration of the eclipse. My grandmother told me about it but then she said that I need not worry about following it, despite the fact that she had practiced all such procedures in her time. Her open mindedness about the changing times left me speechless and utterly grateful. On the other hand, my mother and I shared peals of laughter over the myth that eating spicy food could lead to the baby's hair falling off and flying out of the womb! I made sure to avoid spicy food anyway, but this was to prevent heartburn, and not for any worry about my child's possible baldness due to my dietary decisions!

Even today, our society places far too much value on the boy child. During both my pregnancies, I had women come up to me to assure me that the shape of my belly

Pregnancy and Child Rearing: It's a Family Affair

indicated that I was going to have a boy. People let their imaginations run wild in their attempt to guess the unborn child's gender. If the expecting mother has pimples on her face, it is said that she has a girl child in her womb, who is stealing away her beauty, while glowing skin is associated with boys. A craving for sweet and spicy foods, once again, is thought to signal a baby boy, while sour cravings mean a girl. Needless to say, these so-called signs and indications have no scientific backing at all. Indeed, no external factor in the mother can predict the child's gender. What is more important is this stark preference for the boy child can have a most depressing impact on the mother. After one such social gathering, after having been assured yet again by a group of ladies that I was carrying a boy, I came away rather disconcerted. Abhishek and I talked afterwards about how nobody ever seems to look forward to having a daughter, even though women have shown, time and again, that they are as much of an asset to a family as any of their male siblings. It is a sad reality, and one can only hope that things will continue to change for the better.

As for us, Dania has decreed that she is having a sister this time around. She has made it abundantly clear that we do not have a choice in the matter, for her will needs to be obeyed! In fact, she even told me that on the off chance that a brother *is* born, I should leave him back at the hospital! Baby steps towards gender equality indeed.

12

HAVING IT ALL: A CAREER AND MOTHERHOOD GO HAND IN HAND

Motherhood is a philosophically overwhelming time of life. So much of this journey remains fundamentally indescribable and has to be lived to be understood and appreciated in its entirety. It is simultaneously a universal experience and a unique one. No woman has quite the same experience as her fellow sisters in this journey, or even the same experience in her own consequent pregnancies. But there is something poignant about the first time one becomes a mother. Suddenly, one sees the world through a fresh pair of eyes, from an entirely

Having it All: A Career and Motherhood Go Hand in Hand

new frame of reference. Although pregnancy is a trial by fire, it brings with it a new world of possibilities.

Does this mean that the woman you were before you created this tiny bundle of life has suddenly ceased to exist? Most certainly not! The woman of substance, purpose, and complexity you have grown into over the years continues to thrive. Now, you have an additional layer to add to your fulfillment, through your child. But the old 'you' is only partially hidden, waiting for you to take notice of her and bring her back to life with renewed zest.

It is of vital importance that women imbibe the idea that they were built to add multiple, thriving dimensions to their lives, and that their career can still remain central to them. There are women who choose to focus full-time on motherhood, and I respect and applaud their decision. So long as it is their own choice and of their own volition. However, in our country, we continue to witness an unfortunately large section of the working female population falling out of the workforce post-pregnancy, simply because they have been conditioned to believe that they will not be able to do justice to their roles as mothers if they continue to pursue their careers. Yes, it does take extra effort, planning, determination, grit, and, of course, family support in order to have the best of both worlds. But then again, there is perhaps nothing in life worth having that is not gained through sweat and tears!

Grow Your Baby, Not Your Weight

I am a part of the Indian bureaucratic system, the backbone of governance. It is, to put it mildly, a demanding career. Our jobs require constant firefighting, and the stakes are always high. While most other professions allow for a reasonable period of learning and making mistakes for freshers, we are expected to hit the ground running. The breadth of our duties, and the depth of their consequences are truly very wide. Right from the first posting, given to an officer of the Indian Administrative Service fresh out of training, you deal with a huge team of people working for you. You are entrusted with immense responsibilities from a young age and granted the authority commensurate with your duties. You have the backing of the government resources behind you, and in your office, your word is the law.

As a bureaucrat, I have come to realise that my role is that of a decision-maker. I make the tough choices that impact lives and livelihoods on a daily basis. The results of any work carried out by me and my team are my responsibility; they reflect on my ability to inspire leadership and bring out the best in people. The work that I do has the sanctity of the welfare state, since public service is a joint effort. My team is such that I rarely have to repeat instructions, and results are achieved in record time, no matter what project I take on—and I take pride in that.

But this entire role of boss-lady is redundant the moment I enter my home. There, I have a different little boss waiting

Having it All: A Career and Motherhood Go Hand in Hand

to hand out instructions regarding each of her whims and fancies! The contrast is so painfully stark that it sometimes seems to me that I straddle two worlds at any given time. When Dania came along, older and wiser people advised me, '*Mu pe taala laga lo, ab yeh apne mann se ghar chalayegi.*' And they were right! Dania does not care who her mother is in the professional world, with absolute disregard for the awe, admiration, or trepidation she may inspire in people. Dania wants what she wants, and that's it.

There is a delight in being commanded by a child, which you perhaps enjoy even more if you have a domineering persona and professional reputation. Each time Dania tells me about her latest desire, her wish becomes my command. And what tiny wishes these are, in any case. It takes so little for a child to find joy in life. She wants my time, my hugs and kisses, a few bedtime stories, and the occasional toy. A bowl of chocolates makes her eyes glitter, and a cone of mehendi makes her feel like a princess. It is a blessing that children foster their very own, whimsical little pleasures. The smallest effort, the tiniest show of affection and care on your part wins them over and satisfies their demands. I thank God for making it this way, that parents find it so easy to fulfill their children's innocent demands. For me, my children are my biggest respite from the person that I have to be at work throughout the day. At home, I am happy to be led by their fancies.

Grow Your Baby, Not Your Weight

One of the innate abilities that a mother has is her instinctive ability to juggle roles. Hindu philosophy tells us about the power of Shakti, and the concept of the Mother Goddess has been prevalent in many civilizations throughout the world. This is testimony to the universally acknowledged, but rarely appreciated fact that women are skilled at what modern corporate lingo describes as the ability to 'wear many hats'. This never becomes quite as relevant as when a career-driven woman also becomes a devoted mother. Women have a nurturing side to them, more frequently than men do, and this emerges with renewed vigour upon the arrival of motherhood. This is the primary reason that women are able to be successful professionals and doting mothers at the same time. The world has innumerable examples of this, from Kadambini Ganguly, one of the first women doctors in India, to Justice Leila Seth, the first Chief Justice of an Indian High Court. These are the women I look up to, and, in a humble manner, I hope to count myself among their ranks. And so can any other woman, if she puts her mind to it.

Of course, having it all has never implied doing it all single-handedly. As a mother who is a busy full-time professional, I will never be able to adequately express my gratitude to the veritable team of caregivers who have supported me in my parenting journey. This team has mostly comprised the elder members of my family; my children

Having it All: A Career and Motherhood Go Hand in Hand

have been enormously fortunate to have grown up in the care of family members, not babysitters. I cannot overstate the role my mother, *her* mother, and my mother-in-law have played in parenting my children. Far too often, it was this army of indefatigable superwomen who faced the troubles that make up a huge part of the journey of child-rearing.

Many funny occasions come to mind when I look back to the early years of Dania's life. As a rule, I tend to avoid answering personal phone calls while at work, as I believe that this makes a jarring contrast to the professional atmosphere. One day, I had several meetings scheduled back-to-back that I needed to attend. Most unexpectedly, I found my mother ringing me repeatedly on my phone. After avoiding the calls a couple of times, I decided to answer just to let her know that I was in a meeting and would call once I got free. But the moment I picked up the call, I heard her tired, exasperated voice yelling into the receiver '*Le jaa apne bachche ko, hum se aur nahi sambhalta. Pura ghar fehla kar rakh diya hai!*' ('Come take your child, we cannot manage her any longer. She has turned the entire house upside down!') Amidst my ongoing meeting with 10 odd people, overhearing my mother's voice coming out of my phone and tacitly sympathizing with her, I managed to calm her down for the time being, with the assurance that I would be back home as soon as I possibly could. On my return, I was greeted with a hilarious torrent of complaints from my family. Apparently, our darling offspring had begun her day by breaking a few show pieces, moved on to scattering her food all over the table, and then proceeded to overturn her paint bottles on the floor, colouring it in about ten different shades! No wonder my mother had reached the end of her tether!

It is incidents like these that make a mother learn important lessons in life. That day, I learnt the true meaning of empathy. I cannot imagine the distress my mother must have gone through, but I was overwhelmed with gratitude for her presence in our life. Motherhood has taught me to be kind and compassionate. It has made me more empathetic than I have ever been. When somebody slips up at their job now, I give them the benefit of the doubt. I remind myself that I do not know their story. Perhaps they have a young baby or an ailing parent at home, or perhaps they are having a bad day. Motherhood has taught me patience. The endless questions that you are constantly faced with when bringing up an intelligent toddler makes you reflect on your own intellect, while also increasing your capacity for restraint. This invariably seeps into your professional life as well, so don't be surprised if you become a more respected and admired leader after entering motherhood! And it is not merely virtues that parenthood imparts. Sadhguru, a celebrated contemporary Indian saint, spoke about how the child has an inbuilt ability to extract joy and wonder from

Having it All: A Career and Motherhood Go Hand in Hand

the mundane in life. A child does not need much to be happy. A strangely shaped stone or a particularly sunny day can fill them with pure delight. Children teach us what it means to be alive. Motherhood has made me appreciate the message of the saying, 'the child is father of the man.' My children have taught me how to enjoy life to its fullest, at every step of the way.

A crucial part of becoming a parent is adjusting to having a new, demanding person in the house. Women have a distinct upper hand when it comes to this, since this new person has spent the last nine months inside of them. Moreover, it has been an age-old tradition in most cultures for women to move to their husband's house after marriage, which means an uprooting from a familiar way of life and fitting into a new household altogether. Women have done this with grace and alacrity through the ages, and this flexibility and acceptance of changes allows a mother to make a considerably easier transition from being entirely independent to having a little human dependent on her for its existence.

However, parenthood is only half complete with the mother. The role of the father can never be entirely subsumed by her, no matter how loving and present she is in her children's life. In Indian society, we do not often find fathers being hands-on in the day-to-day business of child rearing. Abhishek did not attend to changing the baby's nappies with any degree of regularity. But the moment his daughter showed any signs of unease, I saw that tough man melt into a bundle of nerves. Every hiccup, and every cough or fever of Dania's made him jittery. The father's role becomes most evident in the emotional support and comfort he provides. It gladdens the mother's heart and lightens the heavy weight of responsibilities on her shoulders. The mother cannot help but feel glad at the attention he gives his children, even if it reduces her own exclusive time spent with her spouse. Such is the magic of motherhood; anything your child receives brings you a large measure of contentment.

Juggling motherhood and a career made me rely on systematic planning more heavily than ever before. When you have a child, you come to accept that the amount of work that is demanded of you at home will have increased manifold. This is regardless of how many people you have helping you to look after your child. At the end of the day, *you* are the mother, and your role in your child's life will never be substituted by any other human being. But your professional growth cannot be allowed to suffer on this account either. The number of hours in a day remain fixed; you simply have to find more efficient ways of managing your work. Routines and timetables are your best friends. Master the art of prioritisation and plan everything to the minutest detail. Do not allow too much to surprise you

Having it All: A Career and Motherhood Go Hand in Hand

or put you off track. With the right systems in place, you can continue on a path embellished with achievements and big wins.

Routines will become equally important in your personal life. It was during my pregnancy, and then as a mother, that I started to place a premium on my health. Earlier, I had gone easy on myself, following erratic eating and sleeping patterns and skipping workouts. But now, it finally dawned on me that my health was the biggest asset I had, which allowed me to live the life of my dreams. Any compromise, and my entire life would be derailed. I became more rigid with my workouts and more precise with my dietary habits than ever before. My children needed me as much as my work did, and I could not afford to let either of them down. Be it my work or my family, I continued to make decisions out of love, and a fierce will to make lives better. This outlook tends to soften the exhaustion, frustrations, and even failures of everyday life.

At this point in life, I have become a juggler par excellence. I have a young daughter and a toddler, and a full-time, extremely demanding career. I have worked throughout my pregnancy, including battling a global pandemic—the coronavirus—from the frontlines of healthcare governance. I have actively monitored renovations in the house, to make independent space for Dania, and extra space for the new baby, and taken care of pre-delivery shopping and cleaning. And I have done all of this with an iron will, a smile etched on my face, even while wondering why on earth we were not given more than twenty-four hours in a day! At the end of the day, I remember the warm little hands that wait to welcome me home and wash away my exhaustion, and the eager mind that talks proudly of what her mummy achieved at work, and all of my tiredness is washed away, with a sense of eternal gratitude for having the life that I do.